BEYOND
SOAP

BEYOND SOAP

The Real Truth About
What You Are Doing to Your Skin and
How to Fix It for a Beautiful, Healthy Glow

———

DR. SANDY SKOTNICKI

with Christopher Shulgan

PENGUIN

an imprint of Penguin Canada, a division of Penguin Random House Canada Limited

Canada • USA • UK • Ireland • Australia • New Zealand • India • South Africa • China

First published 2018

www.penguinrandomhouse.ca

LIBRARY AND ARCHIVES CANADA CATALOGUING IN PUBLICATION

Skotnicki, Sandy, author
Beyond soap : the real truth about what you are doing to your skin and
how to fix it for a beautfiful healthy glow / Sandy Skotnicki.

ISBN 978-0-7352-3360-7 (softcover).—ISBN 978-0-7352-3361-4 (electronic)

1. Skin--Care and hygiene. 2. Cosmetics. 3. Beauty, Personal.
I. Title.

RL87.S56 2018   646.7'26   C2017-904420-6
                                          C2017-904421-4

Book design by Five Seventeen
Cover design by Jennifer Lum
Cover image: DreamPictures/Getty Images
Sensitive skin quiz, pages 18–19, used by permission of Dr. Laurent Misery and
Laboratories Dermatologiques Avène.

Printed and bound in the United States of America

10 9 8 7 6 5 4 3 2

Penguin
Random House
PENGUIN CANADA

To my wonderful parents, Emily and Stan,
who have left this world but are in my thoughts always,
and my beautiful boys, Brandon, Ryan and Spencer

Contents

I've been practising as a dermatologist for 20 years. I'm also on the faculty of the University of Toronto's Department of Medicine. My academic interest is contact dermatitis, or reactions to the things that come into *contact* with the skin. And during my decades in practice I've seen an alarming increase in the number of patients walking into my examining room with a certain kind of skin problem.

The least serious cases complain about sensitive skin. These patients are hyper-aware of whatever's touching them; in fact, they're hyper-aware of their skin. Moving up the scale of severity, there are patients who complain of burning and stinging anytime they put skin products onto themselves, whether the product is moisturizer, soap, sunscreen or something else. Others experience flare-ups due to the friction from their clothing, the wind or sun exposure. We're talking eruptions that range from mild redness to burning or stinging of the face. It might be persistently dry and cracked hands. Or the sensation that the skin or scalp is covered with insects.

Some cases are so severe that patients can't work or sleep because of the constant itch. The reactions affect people's self-esteem and hamper their ability to function. Some feel so ashamed of their rashes that they don't want to go outside. The problems can make many people's lives a living hell.

The type of skin problem I'm talking about, in all its forms, is caused by beauty products. And it's becoming an epidemic. The number of patients I see to treat these reactions has spiked in recent years. I believe my practice is representative of those in developed countries; dermatologists all over the world are noticing increasing numbers.

In 2016, the U.S. Food and Drug Administration made public, for the first time, comprehensive statistics on adverse events related to cosmetic and beauty products. The data trend was alarming in the extreme. For such products as moisturizers, shampoos and conditioners, shaving creams, cleansers, baby products and makeup—the whole of the skincare and beauty product universe, in other words—the FDA registered 291 adverse events in 2013, 436 in 2014, 706 in 2015 and a remarkable 1591 in 2016. Those represent percentage increases of 50 percent, 62 percent and 125 percent in the last three years. You might think these numbers are small relative to population size, but bear in mind, these are events that are *reported* to the FDA. A team from Northwestern University medical school analyzed the data for a study in a major medical journal (*JAMA Internal Medicine*). The study authors noted that the FDA's database "reflects only a small proportion of all events." That is, the actual number of reactions to cosmetic and beauty products is certain to be far higher. Health Canada tracks its own reports on human health and safety concerns related to various types of consumer products—and cosmetics consistently places among the top five reported sectors.

Or consider what's been happening in the last half-century or so with a condition known as eczema—inflamed, scaly, itchy skin. It affects more young people than old. In the 1940s, eczema was relatively rare, affecting just 5 percent of children and comparatively unknown in adults. Today, localities exist where 25 percent of young people suffer from the condition. Adult eczema now affects about 10 percent of adults in the U.S. One interesting thing about eczema is that people with it become more likely to experience other problems, such as asthma and hay fever. A survey that focused on an individual city—Aberdeen, Scotland—found that rates of eczema had increased by three times between 1964 and 1999, while rates of hay fever and asthma had increased by four and five times, respectively. As John McFadden, a dermatologist at London's St. Thomas' Hospital, wrote in the *British Journal of Dermatology*, the skyrocketing eczema rates reflect "a general trend in industrialized countries," and that "during the last decade this increased prevalence has persisted."

The *really* dramatic increase over time has happened with another condition, known as sensitive skin, which is pretty much what it sounds like—skin that is ultra-reactive, intolerant, possibly itchy or otherwise painful, and sometimes, but not always, accompanied by some kind of a rash. The condition is the biggest trend in my practice as well as many others throughout the developed world.

This epidemic troubles some of the world's most respected dermatologists. "The reported prevalence of self-perceived skin sensitivity has increased steadily over time," notes a 2013 article co-authored by the American dermatological legend Howard Maibach. "Knowledgeable, experienced observers agree that the subject is not trivial, causes a great deal of distress, and is more than a cosmetic nuisance or a mere matter of vanity," comments a 2006 article lead-authored by Albert Kligman, the co-inventor of Retin-A.

Reports suggest that 40 percent of people worldwide consider themselves to have sensitive skin. That's a *remarkable* amount. And the research shows that the prevalence can be even higher in

individual countries. One survey revealed that approximately
69 percent of American women self-identified as having sensitive
skin. Nearly 85 percent of women in France claimed to be plagued
by it. And a whopping 91 percent of Italians told researchers that
they suffered from the condition.

Adverse events from beauty products. Skyrocketing rates of eczema.
Huge numbers of people reporting that they have sensitive skin.

What on earth is going on?

This is the 21st century! We have instantaneous access to
nearly any TV show or movie ever filmed. Driverless taxis are
an actual thing! In so many ways, it seems, we're living in the
future—so why does it seem as if we're having more skin
problems than ever? Shouldn't the modern lifestyle have solved
this problem by now?

But here's the thing: *What if that modern lifestyle is part of the
problem?*

———

Evolution invented skin millions of years ago—and until relatively
recently, we've left it to its own devices. Even our great-grandparents
started their lives at a time when most people considered a weekly
bath to be the height of cleanliness.

But then, in the last 70 or so years, we decided that this
wonderful invention *wasn't good enough.* We decided it needed
help. So began the practice of daily showering. The use of soap
several times a day to cleanse the skin. The more-than-daily
application of moisturizers and makeup.

These customs are *incredibly* recent in historical terms.

The bathing and grooming customs of developed societies are a
major contributor to the recent epidemic of skin problems. We
think we're taking care of ourselves by bathing at least every day,
cleansing our faces and bodies multiple times a day, shampooing

several times a week. Not to mention all the other things we do to our skin. But the irony is, many of the things we're doing to *take care* of our skin actually end up *harming* it.

You read that right: The way we're taking care of our skin today is *the wrong approach*.

Whether it's the women in lab coats at the cosmetics counter or the glammed-up influencers on YouTube and Instagram, the conventional wisdom is cleanse, cleanse again, exfoliate, moisturize, protect. *Spend* more money, *buy* more products, *take* more time. No, these things aren't necessary! In fact, most of that advice actually contradicts the academic literature!

What's responsible for the increase in skin problems I described earlier? The modern beauty habits—including our overall obsession with grooming—that are supposed to be taking care of the skin in the first place!

This book isn't another beauty or how-to guide. It's a diagnosis grounded in the latest science that suggests the way we've been taking care of our skin is wrong. As a practising dermatologist, every day I encounter people with major skin reactions. They tend to be astonished when they discover that they may be causing the issue themselves—with a skincare product or the way they wash and take care of their skin.

This book amounts to an objective examination of current beauty and skincare practices, by a medical doctor who's been on the front lines of the battle for skin health for 20 years. The volume you hold in your hands details the latest dermatological science, cutting-edge microbiology and my insider's perspective on the beauty industry to argue that, rather than putting the skin into a cycle of damage and repair—*damaging* with soap, cleansers and treatments, *repairing* with creams and balms—maybe it's better just to sidestep that cycle. To *minimize* such interventions and experience a return to skin health.

The approaches described in this book can help with the following conditions:

- Atopic eczema
- Dandruff
- Dermatitis
- Dry hands
- Dryness or cracking
- Psoriasis
- Reactions to personal-care products
- Rosacea
- Sensitive scalp
- Sensitive skin

But even if you don't suffer from any of these conditions, the principles I outline can help you maintain skin health, fight aging and enhance beauty long into your fifties, sixties, seventies and beyond. I've seen many middle-aged women and men who've struggled for decades with reactive skin. Teenagers spending hundreds of dollars to treat blotchy redness. Elderly people who've tried everything to control their dry, itchy skin. And they've all improved substantially once they've used my approach. Finally, if you just want to understand what is good or bad for your skin from a dermatologist who specializes in ingredients, read this book. The answers will surprise you.

One way to think of it is paleo skincare. Another way? Common sense. However you frame it in your own head, once you've read this book, you'll spend less money on your skin—and it'll look and feel better.

Inside This Book

Chapter 1 gives you a window into my life on the front lines of this epidemic. It also gives you the tools to conduct a self-diagnosis: Are you one of the people I'm describing? Someone who's washing, exfoliating, peeling and cleansing your way into a lifetime of skin problems? Do you in fact have sensitive skin?

Chapter 2 offers you context. How did society reach our bizarre situation, with multibillion-dollar companies selling so many different products to individual consumers that these products can actually end up harming the skin? This history argues that our current mania for cleanliness and skincare products is an incredibly recent phenomenon in terms of human evolution, and represents a corruption of the circumstances the skin has evolved to handle over the course of millions of years.

Chapter 3 is about what's really going on. In it, I explain *why* people in the developed world seem to be experiencing more skin problems than they ever have before. Based on comparative dermatological studies drawn from Amazonian Brazil and the remote Solomon Sea island of Kitava, the chapter observes that people who maintain pre-civilized lifestyles tend to have more diverse skin microbiomes—and cites evidence that overfrequent use of soap, cleansers and some beauty products is causing more problems than they solve.

How did such circumstances evolve? That's the gist of Chapter 4, a description of the sheer size of the skincare industry that worldwide sells an annual $330 billion worth of soaps, cleansers, moisturizers and other skincare products. By visiting skincare companies, I'll make the point that the industry is a business that has been incredibly effective at convincing people to use more skincare products, more frequently—setting up precisely the situation that's causing the sort of skincare reactions I describe in this book.

In Chapter 5, I talk about allergic reactions and how they differ from irritant reactions—and identify which one causes the majority of sensitive-skin reactions. I also provide an in-depth discussion of the problematic ingredients that most frequently cause allergic and irritant reactions.

What to do about all those troubling ingredients, and the reactions they cause? One thing's for sure—you don't just blindly use products that say they're for "sensitive skin," many of which feature ingredients that exacerbate rashes, redness and itchy sensations. Rather, Chapter 6 describes in an easy-to-understand, step-by-step format what I call the product-elimination diet, a protocol for people with reactive skin that represents a reset button for what covers the face, chest, neck, hands and the rest of the body. "Quit using so much stuff" is the gist of the diet, although I'll get into further detail in the chapter. Once you've quit, I provide my preferred list of low-allergenic and fragrance-free products as well as the detailed process of product reintroduction.

Chapters 7, 8 and 9 are guides to skin health. In Chapter 7, I describe how to wash and cleanse the skin in a way that minimizes skin irritation. Chapter 8 is for parents and soon-to-be parents, and details how to care for the skin of new babies, toddlers, children and teens in a way that doesn't set them up for a future of eczema and other problems. Chapter 9 is a guide to minimalist beauty— how to fight aging, preserve skin health and enhance beauty in a way that avoids harm to the skin.

Chapter 10 is about the future of skincare. There's a description of the science-fiction-sounding skincare products that could be released soon, such as a polymer-based "second skin" that still breathes while eliminating wrinkles and DNA-repair enzymes that may begin to repair sun damage with just a couple of applications. The book closes with the prospect of genomic dermatology, which makes it conceivable to imagine DNA technology giving us the capability to design every aspect of human appearance.

How This Book Can Help

This book isn't only for those who have problem skin. Virtually any and all self-described product junkies who follow its minimalist principles will benefit. Within these pages I'll describe the way using too many beauty and skincare products can harm the skin, a phenomenon called cumulative irritation. Ultimately, this book's argument will compel readers to reconsider how they care for their skin and cleanse their bodies. It's an indictment of the way we live today.

I want the book you hold in your hands to represent a wake-up call for our clean-obsessed, product-junkie society. For people to realize that everything they're putting on their skin represents an intervention. A potential problem. People need to realize that the best state for skin is to get it as close as possible to the one it evolved to handle. When we leave skin on its own, it fights wrinkles, staves off aging and acts as armour that protects the body from infection.

Anytime we wash, buff or exfoliate; anytime we moisturize, treat, mist or oil; anytime we slather, spread, hydrate or soften, we're engaging in an intervention that nudges the skin away from its healthiest condition. We've forgotten how wonderful a creation our human bodies are. In particular, we've lost sight of the remarkable abilities possessed by our natural anatomical armour—our skin.

When most men and women in developed societies believe they have sensitive skin, the solution is not another miracle product. Instead, the solution entails moving past the *idea* of miracle products—to return to a time where, as much as possible, we trusted our bodies and the mechanisms they evolved enough that we felt secure leaving skin to its own devices.

1

Do You Have Problem Skin?

The professional woman—I'll call her Jennifer—came into my downtown Toronto dermatology clinic first thing on a Monday morning. I typed her as a lawyer, or a successful advertising executive. She wore a business suit and a pair of conservative heels, and her clothes fit her well. She looked great, in fact, except for one thing.

Her skin looked terrible.

On her cheeks, eyelids and forehead was an outbreak of reptilian-looking scales. The rash started red and transitioned to crusty white flakes, then deepened around her eyes to oozing, open sores. "It's worse on my neck and shoulders," she said, biting her lip to maintain her composure.

She was right: It *was* worse on her shoulders. I felt terrible for her. Scabby patches made it look as though she wore shoulder pads. Raised scarlet bumps climbed up the back of her neck. "Does it hurt?" I asked, and she nodded yes.

"But the worst thing is the itch," she said, rubbing her palm against her shoulders. "I've switched shampoos, tried different sensitive-skin creams and a hypoallergenic cleanser—and nothing works. I went to my doctor—and she referred me to you. Is there *anything* you can do for me?"

Treating rashes like Jennifer's is what I do. It seemed likely to me that Jennifer's rash was caused by one of the very products she was using to *care* for her skin. I see reactions caused by beauty products every day in my practice. As a dermatologist in a major North American city, I'll bet you most days I see three such reactions before my lunch break.

They're *very* common.

So common, in fact, that several years ago I started to get frustrated.

These people—mostly women, some men—were doing this to themselves. Unintentionally, of course. They were listening to the advertising and the suggestions of staff people in the retailers where beauty products are sold. Use *this* cleanser at night, another during the day, another for waking up the skin. Here's a scrub, there's an exfoliator and over *there* is a serum designed to polish your skin. If you heed the rhetoric in the beauty magazines and the YouTube videos, pretty soon you're using more than a dozen beauty products a day. And if you do get a reaction, then a sales clerk will tell you to try something "for sensitive skin," or something labelled "hypoallergenic"—and the problem is, even many of *those* products have irritants and allergens in them.

The skin is protesting against such abuse. That's why I see older men coming in with rashes that climb up and down their shins and teenage girls with inflammation all over their necks and upper backs. That's why I see adults who have struggled all their lives with flare-ups of eczema, rosacea and psoriasis. We're using too many soaps, detergents and beauty products, too frequently.

There are a lot of frustrating things about the skin problems that result. Take sensitive skin. One of the most frustrating things about the condition is that no reliable screening test exists. I can't take a patient blood sample, have it analyzed and then, based on a specific marker, proclaim: Yes, you have sensitive skin! In reality it's completely subjective. In some people, sensitive skin can flare up, present an inconvenience for a couple of days and then disappear without a trace. Others struggle with it for weeks, months and even years.

When I discuss the situation with my patients, sometimes I'll compare the use of beauty products, and the problems that result, to the place that sugar has in the diets of industrialized countries. Which sounds strange on the face of it, but bear with me. As a society, we seem equally addicted to sugar and to beauty products. Another similarity? Like the use of beauty products, and personal grooming in general, sugar is something that became a major component of the human lifestyle comparatively recently, at least in evolutionary terms. In the past few decades people in developed countries have been consuming more of it than they ever have—and our health is suffering in numerous ways as a result. At the start of the 18th century an average adult in England ate about four pounds of sugar a year. At the start of the 19th, the annual consumption of added sugar was up to around 22 pounds—an increase by a factor of more than four. Then fast-forward 200 years to the start of the 21st century, and the average North American consumed about 90 pounds of sugar a year—or more than 20 times what the average English person did three centuries ago. All that sugar has spiked obesity rates, the prevalence of type 2 diabetes and the incidence of inflammation in people across the developed world.

Our habit of using beauty products follows a similar curve. Grooming, along with our use of soap, cleansers and beauty products, has skyrocketed in the last 70 years. The wealthier a country, the more its citizens use these products. We've been washing more, bathing more and applying more beauty products to ourselves in recent decades than we ever have. And just as with our sugar

consumption, this new behaviour is spawning a constellation of
related health problems, most of which affect the skin.

One component of the epidemic in skin problems is sensitive
skin. There are academics, bloggers and beauty experts who question the very existence of this condition. Even some dermatologists would say that "sensitive skin" is little more than a marketing
term—an advertising ploy designed to sell more skincare products. I, too, have my problems with the term. Rather than calling
it "sensitive" skin, I think a better term would be "reactive" or
"intolerant" skin. But there's no doubt that the condition is real.
The people who question the existence of sensitive skin don't see
the reactions that I do on a daily basis. Dermatologists and beauty
experts know that sensitive skin is typically self-induced. But
here's the more important point: The majority of consumers
don't suspect that their condition could possibly be caused by an
organic shampoo or that award-winning face serum made specifically for sensitive skin. Whatever you call it, sensitive skin
exists—and will continue to exist until consumers understand
the real reason why it's happening.

———

In many ways, Jennifer is the classic patient to manifest the sort of
skin problems that plague so many people today. Her income means
she can afford to buy the many different skincare products she uses.
She could have a genetic predisposition for atopic eczema—the
inherited condition I'll discuss in detail in later chapters, which can
set up those who have it with itchy, sensitive and rashy skin,
particularly during flare-ups. Over the years Jennifer has seen many
different experts about her problem—everyone from medical
doctors to the counter person at her local pharmacy to naturopathic
practitioners. She's bought lots of different products that cater to
those with "sensitive skin." And nothing has stopped her reactions.

I arranged for Jennifer to come in for a process called patch testing, which would screen her for an allergy to topical ingredients. But in Toronto, where my practice is located, that meant a three- to six-month wait time.

Jennifer's problem was too serious to wait that long without doing anything. So in the meantime, I prescribed what I call the product-elimination diet, a protocol I use to reset my patients' skin—which I'll describe in Chapter 6. The point is, the product-elimination diet is pretty much the exact opposite of what Jennifer expected. When she'd made the appointment to see me, like most of my patients, she was expecting me to prescribe her a cure-all skin product.

But the majority of people who suffer from the sorts of skin problems I'm describing here don't require an additional *product*. Rather, what they need to do is start subtracting from the number of products they *do* use. Face creams, moisturizing balms, anti-wrinkle gels and age-defying elixirs. They need to bring the skin back to the state of benign neglect that reigned before excessive washing and the invention of skincare.

Just say no to using *stuff*, I told Jennifer. Especially your body wash and shampoo with their multitude of different ingredients.

When I tell patients to stop using most of their skincare products, they look at me as if I'm crazy. Certainly, Jennifer did. They calm down when I tell them that it's only for a short period of time. And here's my logic. As a society we wash way too much, and then we try to limit the damage by applying creams and emulsions that are potentially irritating and allergenic. It would be better if we showered much less frequently than we do today, I told Jennifer. Not too hot, not too long. (Long, hot showers end up drying out the skin.) And once you do get under that falling water, limit how much skin you wash. Most of us would do fine if we didn't use any soap at all. Rather, we should be restricting the shower to a rinse-off, reserving a non-soap cleanser for only those areas where odour can be a problem, such as the groin and underarms.

The products we use on our bodies every day, maybe even many times a day, contain lots of unnecessary ingredients that turn out to be prime candidates for skin irritation and potential allergy. Jennifer certainly didn't need to be using so many products.

In fact, few of us do.

NORTH AMERICA'S TOP FIVE SKIN DISEASES

1. *Acne vulgaris*: also known as acne
2. *Fungal skin disease*: includes athlete's foot, jock itch, ringworm and yeast infections
3. *Eczema*: also called atopic eczema, a group of medical conditions that cause inflamed or irritated skin
4. *Pruritus*: itching skin
5. *Impetigo*: skin infection that usually appears as red sores on the face and mainly affects infants and children

A Changed Woman

Three weeks later, Jennifer returned to my office for a follow-up appointment. She smiled as soon as she saw me. "It's gone!" she said.

Jennifer showed me her shoulders, and lifted the hair off the back of her neck to show me her nape. All of it was healthy skin. The rash had completely disappeared. "I thought you were crazy," she said. "But you know what? What you suggested worked."

Allergy testing later revealed just what I'd suspected. Jennifer had been having an allergic reaction to a specific ingredient in her shampoo—a preservative called methylisothiazolinone, or MI.

"Dr. Skotnicki, you fixed me!" Jennifer exclaimed.

I hear similar sentiments from other patients all the time.

Jennifer's was an extreme case—a true allergic reaction. The majority of sensitive-skin cases are caused by using too many products, and poor product labelling, which then lead to reactive or intolerant skin. I just wish I could get to these patients before they lather, buff and rub themselves into the problems such interventions cause.

At this point, many readers may be wondering whether they're setting themselves up for skin problems. Are you on the road to a reaction like Jennifer's? Or perhaps something less severe that's preventing your skin from achieving the health that it otherwise might?

Many of my patients conform to certain types. There are the women who stay attuned to the latest trends in beauty and fashion. They're always on the lookout for new products to use. They spend time in salons. They troll the mall for interesting new makeup or other products. And they feel a little frisson of excitement whenever a stylist, retail clerk or social media maven suggests something new. At home, this type has a vanity somewhere that's full of old products—half-used shampoos and conditioners, exfoliating masks, chemical peels. I call this sort of patient the aforementioned *product junkie.*

Another classic type in my practice is something like the opposite. Usually men, these are *frequent exercisers* who need to look good at work. Maybe they're in finance, or in sales. Probably they wear suits to the office. And at some point through the course of the day, they're exercising. And showering after the workout. Even though they may use only a handful of beauty products— soap and shampoo, conditioner, deodorant and maybe a hair gel— these people are showering around a dozen times a week, and likely soaping all over their bodies when they do. Over time, this consistent assault on the external layers leads to a rash, or some kind of worse skin reaction.

A third type I often see in my practice is the *organic friend of the earth.* Male or female, these are people who may have already experienced skin reactions to beauty products, possibly due to a pre-existing skin condition. Their history has made them suspicious of anything that has an ingredient with a chemical-sounding name. They opt for natural products often created by alternative beauty companies, avoiding things like parabens or such chemical surfactants as sodium lauryl sulphate. But although opting for natural and organic is a smart strategy when it comes to the food you put in your mouth, it's not always best for the things you put on your skin, particularly when natural fragrances are among some of the most allergenic and irritating substances out there.

I'm not judging any of these types of patients. In fact, there are aspects of me in each one. I like my beauty products, am a frequent exerciser, have reactive skin and also consider myself a friend of the earth. Luckily, I'm also a dermatologist who sees terrible skin reactions every day. My experiences have taught me a set of principles that allow me to minimize my own skin reactivity and enhance my skin health—and I'll get to those later in the book.

If you recognize yourself in one of the three types I've outlined, or simply believe you may be headed for a skin reaction, I'll leave you with a little quiz. One way to ascertain whether you suffer from sensitive skin was pioneered in 2014 by the French dermatologist Laurent Misery, who established a 100-point scale of severity. If you have a piece of paper handy, you can conduct the questionnaire yourself. Here it is, in step-by-step form.

1. Score from zero to 10, with 10 being the maximum irritation, your degree of overall skin irritation in the past three days.
2. Now score the severity you've experienced for each of the following sensations, again over the past three days:
   a. Burning
   b. General discomfort

  c. Hot flashes

  d. Itching

  e. Pain

  f. Sensations of heat

  g. Tautness

  h. Tingling

3. At this point you should have a score out of 90. One score for overall discomfort, followed by a score out of 10 for each of the eight sensations in question two. Finally, give yourself a score from zero to 10 on the redness of your skin over the past three days.

Now add up the scores you've awarded yourself. The highest total possible is 100. Dr. Misery, the dermatologist who pioneered the scale, led a team that conducted the questionnaire with about 3000 patients who had previously complained of sensitive skin. The average score was 36.49 out of 100, with Dr. Misery suggesting that anyone who scored higher than 20 would qualify as suffering from sensitive skin.

If you *don't* have a sheet of paper and just want the simplest way to determine whether you have sensitive skin, ask yourself the following questions:

1. Do you regularly experience a burning or tingling sensation, skin tightness or other irritation on your face, hands or the skin anywhere else on your body?

2. Do you break out easily in a rash or experience redness or flushed skin due to changes in temperature, brightness, wind strength, moisture content of the air or other environmental triggers?

3. Does exposure to cosmetic products, such as makeup, cleanser, soap, moisturizer, sunscreen or shampoo, provoke the emergence of a rash or any other skin reaction?

4. Does exposure to fragranced products, such as hand soap, perfumes or colognes, insect repellents or styling gels, provoke the emergence of a rash or any other skin reaction?

If you answered yes to any of the above questions, then you likely have some degree of sensitive skin—and could benefit from the treatments, techniques and information contained in the rest of this book.

2

The Cleanliness Obsession

It happens a couple of times a week. A patient comes into my office with a nasty rash. "I've been cleaning it," the patient explains as we examine the bumpy, irritated skin. "But even though I'm washing it several times a day, it doesn't get any better."

The problem, I explain to the patient, isn't that the rash has become dirty. The problem is, you're washing *too much*. You're irritating the skin with the cleanser you're using, which creates the skin sensitivity and the rash. So no matter how much you wash, the thing doesn't go away, because *the washing is the cause*.

As a society we've become obsessed with cleanliness as a panacea for all our ills. One of the reasons my patients wash so much is that they think it keeps them healthy—and beautiful. Wash, cleanse, scrub, exfoliate, disinfect—whatever the term we use, we're doing too much of it, and that fact is contributing to this epidemic of sensitive skin.

The trick is to differentiate between hygiene and cleanliness. I like the thinking here of Dr. Sally Bloomfield, a U.K. expert in the prevention of infectious disease, who has called for us to separate the two concepts of hygiene and cleanliness. *Hygiene*, she says, involves practices required to protect us from infectious diseases. Washing your hands after you've used the subway to return home from work is an example of a *hygienic* practice—because you're getting rid of the germs you touched on the escalator railing, the subway straps, the buttons you pressed on the fare-card dispenser.

In contrast, Bloomfield says, *cleanliness* is the absence of dirt, the feeling of freshness, the desire for social acceptability: "We thus need to distinguish between routines associated with cleanliness, in the sense of absence of dirt, appearance, social acceptability and freshness, and those practices required to protect us from infectious disease."

The washing practices that keep us healthy and hygienic are a lot less rigorous than the washing processes we've been socialized into thinking keep us clean. In fact, we've become so obsessed with cleanliness that it's making us unhealthy. In many cases, we're washing our bodies so much that we're damaging the protective layer the body uses to ward off harm from the elements. In the name of cleanliness, we're exposing our skin to products that are harming what they're supposed to improve.

How did we get to the point where we feel dirty if we don't lather the body in soapsuds at least once a day? Our personal hygiene and skincare routines have changed dramatically in the last 70 years. For millennia, in fact for vast swaths of mammalian evolution, most of us didn't do much at all to our skin.

The genus *Homo* first evolved in Africa 2.5 million years ago. Two million years ago, humankind spread from Africa to Eurasia. And 200,000 years ago, *Homo sapiens* evolved in East Africa. It wasn't until 70,000 years ago that *sapiens* spread from Africa. We settled in North America just 16,000 years ago. The agricultural revolution, which saw us domesticating plants and animals for the first time, happened just 12,000 years ago. Not until 5000 years ago did there come the first kingdoms, written languages and use of currency for transactions.

Now consider that the skin *predates all of that.* It's remarkable to think about, but the basic principles of the way the skin works, just like the basic principles of other important biological organs like the heart or the brain, predate the development of humanity. By the time the genus *Homo* evolved, the principle of evolution had already worked out the general gist of how to keep mammalian insides from spilling out into the world in a way that protected important interior stuff, like muscles and blood, while also conveying information about the outside world to the brain *and* being permeable to things like water, oil and salt.

So skin's been around for more than 2.5 million years. And for the vast majority of that time, we didn't do much to it. Maybe we smeared some mud on our faces, the better to hide in the underbrush as we stalked whatever land animal happened to be that afternoon's prey. Maybe we plunged ourselves into a river or lake on a sweltering hot day. But most of us were too busy determining how to put food into our mouths to concentrate much on whether our skin ever "radiated a youthful glow."

And you know what? Our skin did pretty well. The epidermis existed in a state of benign neglect. Skin cells died, flaked off, became dust. Bacteria colonized the skin until we hosted an average of a million microbes per square centimetre, with a whopping 158 different bacterial species existing on the average palm. We gave off a certain body odour, sure, but that scent included pheromones that helped one sex attract the other in such a way that we propagated our species.

So how did we develop our current ideas of hygiene and cleanliness—and how did things get mixed up to the extent that they have? Few people know more about the earliest development of the topic than Valerie Curtis, director of the Hygiene Centre at the London School of Hygiene & Tropical Medicine. In her research, Curtis describes as "hygienic" any behaviour that helps to "avoid the risk of being invaded by parasites." In fact, she argues that hygienic behaviour far predates the evolution of humans. Curtis believes that these behaviours date back to at least 600 million years ago, with creatures as basic as nematode worms avoiding disease-causing bacteria named *Bacillus thuringiensis*.

Curtis has found that many other basic earthbound creatures demonstrate hygienic behaviour. Ants, she writes, "groom them-selves to remove fungal pathogens" and isolate other ants that are either dead or diseased. Even undersea creatures—like certain types of lobsters, about as different a species from human as it's possible to get on earth—will avoid other lobsters showing signs of sickness.

All vertebrates engage in the sort of grooming actions we associate with hygiene, Curtis believes. She cites the way bullfrog tadpoles can avoid other tadpoles that exhibit signs of a particular sickness. Most mammals, fish and birds groom themselves to remove parasites that live on the skin or in scales and feathers. And everything from birds to grazing animals like sheep, reindeer and caribou tend to take steps to avoid mixing their food with any bodily waste.

Of course, no one *taught* such creatures these behaviours. Rather, the customs *evolved*, or, as Curtis nicely puts it, "the long gradual process of evolution was their teacher." Genes that contributed to "good strong hygiene instincts" were able to multiply, while the genes that contributed to behaviour that tended to infect creatures with disease selected themselves out. Good hygiene seems to be an innate, evolutionary urge for all sorts of animals.

Of course, humans display this evolutionary urge as much as any other creature. If not more. As a society we have a strong impulse to wash and clean. *The problem is*, we've gone too far.

"Disgust of dirt is a part of human nature," Curtis writes, hypothesizing that at its core, "disgust is what humans call the urge to avoid disease-relevant stimuli." To test the hypothesis, Curtis designed a survey that appeared on the website of the British

Broadcasting Corporation. The survey asked participants to rate how disgusting they found a series of photos. The study was completed by 40,000 people from around the globe. And in general, images with "disease relevance" were rated as more disgusting than those without any connection to disease at all. For example, a photo of clean, burned skin tended to be rated as less disgusting than a photo of an infected abrasion.

Curtis and her fellow researchers concluded that "disgust is probably common to all humans in all cultures, and that it serves to help us avoid those things that were associated with risk of disease in our evolutionary past. Disgust is thus the name we give to the motivation to behave hygienically."

If Curtis's thinking is correct, then even the earliest of human beings likely exhibited some sort of grooming behaviour. Probably the earliest men and women picked fleas and other parasites off their fellow humans. They likely emptied their bladders and bowels some distance away from the shelters where they slept and ate. And the earliest humans likely avoided other humans who displayed evidence of infection. They also probably avoided the bodies of dead humans, which can harbour many types of different diseases.

At some point, hygienic customs developed *beyond* the instinctive behaviours required to minimize contact with the stuff that makes us sick. We progressed to actions designed to make us look better and more attractive to potential mates.

It's difficult to establish exactly when this happened. Curtis mentions cave paintings that depict beardless men, which suggests some sort of an effort to remove facial hair. Was this intended to make the men more attractive? Or simply to remove fleas? The answer is lost to history. Neanderthals used seashells as tweezer-like tools, Curtis says, possibly for the same sort of hair-removal sessions that we conduct today. She notes that archaeologists have found ivory combs that date back to Egypt of 3200 BCE. Digs in the locations of ancient cities in the Indus River basin of Pakistan and India have turned up constructs thought to be toilets and drain facilities—dating back to 3000 BCE.

So when did we start to *wash*? That's a tough practice to date. Much of what we know about ancient cultures comes from the tools those cultures left behind. Beyond soap, the practice of washing requires few tools. And soap biodegrades. So although it's possible that some caveman or -woman, somewhere, combined ash and animal fat to create the most basic form of soap, it's impossible to know for sure.

Some accounts have the first definitive examples of cleansing behaviour occurring in Greek and Roman societies, dating back to the sixth century BCE and featuring the use of oil and a scraper known as a *strigil*. The Romans also used plumbing and toilets. Varying reports place the earliest definitive use of soap in either Babylonian or Phoenician societies, depending on which source you believe. Archaeologists found a soapy substance in earthenware jars discovered at an excavation dated to ancient Babylon, around 2800 BCE, nearly 5000 years ago. But the purpose of the soap is lost to history.

———

Perhaps the soap cleaned food stains from garments. Perhaps the soap sloughed off blood and fat from the skin of someone butchering an animal. But today we engage in a daily shower even when we haven't been butchering animals. And we don't limit our grooming behaviours to showering. We scrub and we buff, we exfoliate and we polish. We cleanse and we loofah and we lather. Today many of us shower at least daily not out of a need to stay healthy, but rather out of an obsessive desire to achieve the insane levels of cleanliness that society suggests is required.

So how did we get here? The situation may have started around the time of the Ebers Papyrus, a 20-metre-long Egyptian scroll that dates from 1500 BCE. It's one of the oldest preserved medical documents. Said to have been found with a mummy in an ancient cemetery near the Egyptian city of Thebes, the scroll is a comprehensive textbook summarizing the extent of Egyptian medical knowledge. Some of the writing we would dismiss outright today, including spells and incantations intended to ward off disease. As a form of birth control it suggests smearing mashed-up dates, acacia and honey on wool and inserting the whole thing into the vagina—which isn't something this medical doctor would ever recommend.

But the scroll also correctly identifies the heart as the centre of the blood supply. It describes the mixing of animal and vegetable fats with alkaline salts to form a substance—which would have been a rudimentary soap—that can be used to treat skin diseases and remove dirt from the skin.

As Curtis points out, religions of all sorts seem to have played a major role in the association of soap with purity, which leads directly to the daily all-over washing that's so common in contemporary society. Ancient Mesopotamian society featured a ritual known as *kippuru*, which saw a flour paste smeared onto the skin and then wiped off. The ritual is the source of the word "purification." Meanwhile, Hindu scripture counselled *its* followers to avoid what it called the body's 12 impurities, which included oily exudations, semen, blood, urine, feces, mucus, ear wax, phlegm, tears, eye sleep and sweat—one of the earliest conceptions I can find that conceive of the body's natural substances as "dirty." But Hindu religion isn't alone in that type of thinking.

The Bible features many examples that associate "cleanliness as next to Godliness," with the Old Testament book of First Corinthians preaching that everyone from thieves to drunkards and adulterers can become "righteous" if they are "washed." Similarly, the Muslim Koran points out that God loves those who "keep themselves clean."

Indoor plumbing was common in a handful of pre-modern civilizations, from Greek and Roman bathhouses to East Asian

dynasties to the cultures of the Indus river valley. What prevented
the bathhouse culture from making it to the Europe of the Industrial
Revolution? Just a little something called the Black Death.

The plague originated in European rodent populations and
spread to humans through bites from fleas that fed on both rats and
humans. It killed 8 out of every 10 people afflicted, resulting in the
deaths of 50 million Europeans between 1346 and 1353,
approximately 60 percent of the continent's total population. And
one long-lasting effect of the plague was a European fear of water,
which was incorrectly thought to have spread the disease. For
centuries afterward, people on the continent cleansed by wiping
themselves with dry cloths, using water only minimally.
Consequently, Europeans would become legendary for their
powerful stench when they visited Arabia or the Far East.

Grooming for the Europeans didn't mean *washing*; rather, it
meant using powerful perfumes to mask odour. Soap was produced
in just a few European cities, such as Marseilles, France, and Castille,
Spain. And according to Geoffrey Jones, a professor of business
history at Harvard and the author of *Beauty Imagined: A History of
the Global Beauty Industry*, Western society had a "limited demand"
for soap until the 1860s. "The craft of making soap, like perfume,
was ancient, but so was people's refusal to use it," writes Jones.

Things began to change with the advent of germ theory—
the advance in medical science that identified infection as being
caused by tiny creatures that can be killed by washing with soap.
In the 1670s in the Dutch Republic, the father of microbiology,
Antonie van Leeuwenhoek, used a compound microscope to peer
at the tissue scraped from between his teeth—and found, upon
high magnification, something he called animalcules—bacteria.

It would take several hundred more years, until the second part
of the 19th century, for the idea to spread that those bacteria might
be responsible for disease. One of the primary figures helping

things move along was Ignaz Semmelweis, an obstetrician who worked at Vienna's General Hospital. In 1847, he noticed that women who delivered babies with the help of doctors and medical students were contracting fevers, while those who delivered with the help of midwives were not. In 1846, for example, the doctor-staffed clinic featured a death rate five times greater than the midwife-staffed clinic. We now know that what was giving the women fevers was a bacterial infection of the uterus or genital tract, known as childbed fever, contracted after giving birth to a child. According to an article in *The New England Journal of Medicine*, "It was the single most common cause of maternal mortality, accounting for about half of all deaths related to childbirth."

The infection caused women agony at a vulnerable time. It also became a major preoccupation of pregnant women, the thing many of them fixated on amid their overall birth-related anxiety. Semmelweis was intent on determining why so many women in the obstetric ward were dying of the disease while comparatively few died in the *midwife* ward. His epiphany occurred after the death of one of his physician mentors.

During an autopsy, the mentor had been pricked with a scalpel that had been cutting through a cadaver. Semmelweis noticed that the fever that killed the physician had symptoms similar to childbed fever.

Because Semmelweis's hospital, Vienna General, was a teaching hospital, the doctors and students in the deadly obstetric ward frequently examined cadavers, with their bare hands, then used those same hands to examine pregnant women. (The midwives in the safe birth ward did not examine cadavers.) What if, Semmelweis thought, the "cadaverous particles" on the physicians' hands were causing the women's bacterial infection?

The solution, he decided, was to have the physicians *wash their hands*. They washed after they touched the cadavers, before they touched the genitals of the pregnant women—and the death rate in the obstetric ward dropped from 11.4 percent to just 1.3 percent.

Unfortunately, the medical community failed to comprehend the importance of Semmelweis's ideas. His fellow doctors ridiculed his theory and rejected the notion that handwashing could reduce infection. Increasingly obsessed with convincing his fellow doctors, Semmelweis developed a severe drinking problem. In 1865, seven years after he published his theory, he was committed to a mental institution, where he was beaten by guards and died. The hospital where Semmelweis worked returned to doing things the old way—and mothers' mortality rates jumped in the doctor-staffed obstetric ward.

BEAUTY THROUGH THE AGES

ANCIENT EGYPT

Aristocrats who lived thousands of years ago around the Nile engaged in elaborate beauty regimens, according to Mark Tungate's *Branded Beauty*. Egyptian bathing involved washing with an early form of soap made by blending oil with natron, a mixture of sodium carbonate, sodium bicarbonate and salt found naturally in dry North African lake beds. The final part of the bath involved an exfoliating treatment that used clay and ash. After the bath came a massage with an ointment of turpentine and incense, intended to mask body odour. Then came makeup.

Nile-area women pioneered the first eyeliner, kohl, which amounted to powdered lead sulphite mixed with animal fat. Aristocratic Egyptians stored it in a case that also contained an appropriate tool for application, such as a small bone or stick—likely the earliest compacts. Wrinkle-reducing foundation consisted of powdered alabaster, salt and natron mixed with honey. Women applied powdered ochre to the skin to create a golden appearance, and used such substances as charcoal and malachite for eye shadow.

The Egyptian beauty regimen also involved elaborate early versions of manicures and pedicures that employed rudimentary tweezers and razors created from painstakingly sharpened bronze. Fingernails were polished with henna, and hair was tamed with combs, then plaited or pressed to the scalp with metallic headbands and hairpins made from ivory.

ANCIENT GREECE

In contrast to the elaborate beauty rituals used by the Egyptians to the south, the Greek women of male-dominated Sparta and Athens weren't allowed to use makeup unless they were prostitutes. "The Greeks believed that beauty lay in natural harmony rather than the application of face paint," Tungate writes. There was one loophole: The women were allowed to wear minimal makeup on their wedding night.

Around 600 years before Christ, according to Tungate, Oriental beauty techniques filtered into Greek society. In this era, women began to whiten their skin. Some used powdered chalk; others, something known as ceruse—a mineral called lead carbonate, or white lead. Meaning, it actually contained the element lead, which is poisonous. When applied to the skin over time, ceruse would cause hair loss, headaches, brain damage and even death. This marked possibly the first time that women sacrificed long-term body function for short-term beauty gains. It certainly wouldn't be the last.

TANG DYNASTY

Approximately 1300 years ago, as the remains of the Greco-Roman civilization were disintegrating half a world away, the Tang Dynasty presided over China from one of the world's most populous cities— while also employing some of history's most elaborate beauty regimens.

Women applied white face powder, rouged their cheeks and yellowed their foreheads with skin paint made of herbs and flowers. The next step involved painting on eyebrows in a fascinatingly

diverse series of shapes that changed with the year's fashions—
everything from narrow arcs to thick, moonlike orbs set on the
mid-forehead. Rouge was applied to the lips to make them appear
full and, in some cases, pursed. A pair of red dots on either side of
the lips, known as *mian-ye*, indicated whether the woman was
menstruating. Finally, an ornament of foil, paper or fishbone would
be glued to the middle of the forehead, and hair would be bundled
up into an elaborate, gravity-defying shape.

Twenty years later, in France, Louis Pasteur and his
contemporaries popularized the germ theory of disease, which
holds that tiny organisms can make us sick—unless we halt the
spread of disease by washing our hands, among other hygienic
behaviours. Poor Semmelweis had been right all along. Quite
rightly, germ theory would lead to public health campaigns that
encouraged the use of soap and water to wash. Germ theory also
contributed to government investments in infrastructure that led to
indoor plumbing—which did a lot to increase the human lifespan
by making it easier to clean kitchen surfaces and floors as well as
dirty laundry. The problem is that the hygienic behaviour that
evolved out of germ theory grew into an obsession with cleanliness
that persists to this day. So what happened?

One thing is certain: Advertising helped.

Before germ theory came along, few North American or
European homes featured indoor plumbing. Bathing frequency seems
to have entailed the occasional warm-weather dip in a pond, stream
or river. The water-supply techniques that brought most Westerners
showers and baths didn't begin to develop until the rapid growth in
urban population engendered by the Industrial Revolution. "As their
populations expanded, London, Paris, New York City, Boston, and
other large Western cities began to develop squalid slums whose
inhabitants had no access to clean water," writes Geoffrey Jones. A

wave of epidemics—flu, typhus, cholera—ensued in the middle of
the 19th century, prompting local governments to fund public
infrastructure projects that first brought clean water to homes.

It took a series of wars to bring the benefits of hygiene to the
masses, according to Jones. Florence Nightingale saved many lives
in the Crimean War of the 1850s simply by washing wounded
soldiers with soap, and the American Civil War saw the North
founding a Sanitary Commission that encouraged washing with
soap. "War may be a dirty business, but it was good for the soap
business," Jones writes. The efforts of Nightingale and the Sanitary
Commission led to a popular movement, known as the Sanitarians,
which campaigned for regular washing.

A 2012 paper from the International Scientific Forum on Home
Hygiene (ISFHH) places the beginning of the increase in bathing
frequency in the U.S. and U.K. somewhere between 1890 and 1915.
As a result of higher cleanliness standards, the authors write,
legislation was enacted in the U.K. requiring local governments to
provide bathing and laundry facilities for people who didn't have
them in their own homes. And before the First World War, most
American homes didn't have indoor plumbing either.

Well into the 20th century most Europeans considered bathing
a *weekly*, rather than daily, routine. In England, according to the
ISFHH, "home bathing and laundering became a social norm in
the years immediately before and after World War II; in the U.S. it
might have happened slightly earlier." The Forum believes that
in-home stand-up showers began to be installed in middle-class
American homes somewhere between the 1940s and 1960s, "with
the proportion of American homes with bathtubs and/or showers
increasing from 61% in 1940 to 87% in 1960."

But why did Westerners feel the need to install these showers?
That's where the advertising comes in. Even as British and American
homes began to feature indoor plumbing, soap was cheap, widely

available and mostly unbranded. Bathing frequency increased in parallel to the development of a consumer-products industry—and the growth of the advertising agencies that sold its products.

The firm that did the most to create a mass market for soap was a Cincinnati company called Procter & Gamble, founded in 1837. One of the early drivers of its business was candles. It also sold unbranded cakes of soap. When the wide availability of oil lamps began depressing candle sales, P&G turned to a new business, and in 1879 debuted a product called Ivory Soap. The product featured some innovative elements. Individually wrapped, and made with palm and coconut oils rather than the more traditional olive oil, Ivory Soap was so pure, the advertising said, that it floated on water.

Another innovation was the marketing. In the early 1880s, most American magazines, if they featured any advertising at all, marketed patent medicines with dubious claims. But according to Jones, a member of the second generation of P&G's owners, Harley Procter, invented a marketing strategy based on advertising in magazines, including the best-selling title of them all, *The Century Illustrated Monthly Magazine*. The advertising emphasized the brand, Ivory, rather than the manufacturer, P&G, and featured academics attesting to the quality of the soap. Sales ascended so steeply that P&G built a new factory outside Cincinnati that could manufacture two million boxes of soap a year. By 1890, P&G was America's foremost soap maker. The impetus for Ivory's success did not go unnoticed; by the early years of the 20th century the soap industry was among America's largest advertisers, according to Jones.

Although P&G had domestic competition, such as Colgate and Palmolive, it was the Cincinnati company's British counterpart, Lever, that became the other global powerhouse of the soap industry, according to Jones. Founded by a grocer named William Lever from Lancashire in northern England, the company's initial success derived from its use of pine kernel oil to make soap that lathered more easily than market competitors. Lever's first branded soap, Sunlight, debuted in 1885. He entered the American market the following decade, and in 1896 launched Lifebuoy soap, the first antibiotic soap brand, which contained carbolic acid. Another big hit was Lux brand soap flakes. By 1914, the company was selling half the soap bought in Britain.

Both Lever and P&G advertised heavily. "The emergence of soap, and the practice of washing with water, as a symbol of social status and of the moral superiority of Western civilization, would have seemed implausible at the start of the nineteenth century," writes Jones. "Once societal attitudes towards hygiene had begun to shift, the soap companies drove the growth of demand both through advertising and the creation of mass-production facilities."

By the dawn of the 20th century, soap was no longer marketed exclusively as a tool to aid human hygiene. Advertising had helped transform the one-time commodity into the first widely available beauty product—the use of which was required to maintain an appearance acceptable to polite society. Sales climbed as a result. In 1904 the United States manufactured about 700,000 tons of soap; by 1919 that figure had more than doubled to 1.7 million tons.

Contributing to the rise was the sort of marketing that the advertising agency J. Walter Thompson conducted with a Jergens brand, Woodbury Facial Soap. In a campaign that ran in such women's magazines as *Ladies' Home Journal*, the agency linked the use of Woodbury's to the development of what would now be called a woman's "sex appeal."

"So few people really understand the skin," one 1911 Woodbury advertisement begins. "Whatever the condition that is keeping your skin from being beautiful, it can be changed. . . . Is your skin colorless, sallow, coarse textured and excessively oily? Are there little rough places in it that make it look scaly when you powder? . . . The best way to make this new skin so strong and healthy . . . is by proper cleansing with a soap carefully prepared to suit the nature of the skin."

The ad then advises a beauty treatment: Lather up a bar of Woodbury's with warm water and then work the "antiseptic lather" in an "upward and outward motion" into the skin. "Rinse with warm water, then with cold," the copy counsels. "Then rub your face for several minutes with a lump of ice."

Never mind that the harsh cleansing regimen was far more likely to dry out your skin and make your skin problems *worse*. After just five years of the campaign, in 1916, sales of Woodbury's increased sixfold. These types of advertising, not just for soap but also for tooth powder, mouthwash, shaving creams and antiperspirants, created a sense that certain aspects of the human condition—the odour that exists in mouths, say, or those emanating from underarms and other body parts—were shameful and distasteful. In fact, the human body itself was inherently dirty, the new advertising implied. "The right soap promised to signal social respectability, and even to transform one's romantic life," Jones points out.

The market was growing, but by the time of the First World War it remained by no means saturated. According to Kathy Peiss's *Hope in a Jar*, only one-fifth of Americans used any toiletries or cosmetics in 1916. But beginning in the post–Second World War United States, and continuing all over the world today, we've been inundated with advertising for soaps and cleansers, serums and balms, all of them designed to cure our every insecurity or body-image issue. It's not all the fault of the consumer-products companies or the advertisers. They are, after all, attempting to provide us with solutions to pre-existing human insecurities. Nevertheless, it's hard to deny that our instinct to wash long ago passed from what's required for health and hygiene into a full-blown cultural obsession.

———

According to a July 2014 survey by the market research company Euromonitor, those in the industrialized world now shower an average of once a day. But with their daily workouts and demanding social lives, the sort of urban professionals who predominate in *my* practice average a lot more than that.

The result? A society that may be more obsessed with personal hygiene and grooming than at any other time in human history. The point I hope you'll glean from this chapter is that through most of history, most people didn't cleanse or moisturize—and their skin did fine, thank you very much. Our obsessive washing today has more to do with the advertising industry's ability to play on our insecurities than any health-related need to ensure the hygiene of the skin.

In fact, I believe that Western culture is now caught in a destructive cycle. We start with consumer products like soap, shower gel and shampoo, which strip the natural oils from our skin, removing precisely what it needs to keep it protected from the environment. Then we mitigate the damage by slathering our bodies with moisturizers and other stuff we'd never need if we didn't wash too much in the first place. In turn, overwashing and overfrequent product use are creating new problems, including sensitive skin—and I'll describe exactly how that's happening in Chapter 3.

Damaging Our Body's Natural Armour

If the history of skincare shows one thing, it's that our era is an aberration—that most times throughout history, most people, with the exception of high society, didn't think much of skincare at all. So let's conduct a thought experiment. What was skin like *before* contemporary civilization? Before department stores and pharmacies stocked their shelves with dozens of brands of skin creams, soaps and cleansers?

A host of academic studies have attempted to answer this question. They've tended to focus on acne, and in general they've looked at isolated communities that have tended to follow a non-industrial way of life. It's a great idea. How do you learn about how the contemporary lifestyle affects the skin? You ferret out communities that don't live the contemporary lifestyle.

Acne is nearly as prevalent in developed societies as sensitive skin. As a dermatologist with three teenage sons, I'm as conscious of that as anyone. Acne afflicts between 40 and 50 million Americans of diverse ages—not just teenagers. One study that looked at the prevalence in adults over the age of 25 found that 54 percent of women and 40 percent of men reported some degree of acne. The rates are

even higher for adolescents. In the United States, approximately
85 percent of people between the ages of 12 and 24 experience at
least minor acne. Other studies based on populations in such developed societies as Scotland, New Zealand and Australia place the
prevalence at between 79 and 95 percent of 16- to 18-year-olds.

What's the prevalence of acne in societies that *don't* subscribe
to the modern way of life? Some of the most interesting studies
attempting to answer that question date back many decades, when
a greater part of the world remained comparatively unaffected by
the lifestyles of industrialized nations. For example, back in 1951,
Dr. Otto Schaefer, a German physician, moved to the Canadian
north at the age of 32 to work with the Inuit. He learned the Inuit
language, travelled by dog sled and researched the health and nutrition of an isolated population only then adopting modern customs.
Schaefer saw that Inuit who followed the industrialized lifestyle
tended to grow to heights one to two inches higher than their ancestors. Another thing Schaefer noticed? Increasing rates of acne.

A similarly isolated society that integrated with Western lifestyles
around the same period inhabited the island of Okinawa in the South
China Sea. Before the Second World War, the community pursued a
rural way of life—and, not incidentally, apparently experienced no acne.

Both of these communities were mentioned in a well-known
dermatological study published in the *Archives of Dermatology* in
2002. The study also reports on an effort to examine nearly 10,000
schoolchildren aged 6 to 16 years in a rural, non-industrialized
region of Brazil, finding that just 2.7 percent of them had acne.
What's more, lower rates of acne than those common in the
industrialized world were reported among non-industrialized
societies in Peru and South Africa, according to the study.

But the researchers for this *Archives of Dermatology* paper wanted
to conduct their own observations. One of the study authors, Staffan
Lindeberg, travelled to a remote island named Kitava in the

Solomon Sea, northeast of Papua New Guinea. Residing in villages of between 20 and 400 people, Kitavan islanders lived on what they could harvest from the sea and the soil. Lindeberg, an MD, visited every house on the island, all 494 of them, and conducted physical examinations on 1200 residents aged 10 or older. He looked for acne, or evidence of acne scarring, by examining male subjects' face, chest and back and female subjects' face and neck.

The results were pretty remarkable. "Not a single papule, pustule, or open comedone was observed in the entire population," the paper reports. ("Comedone" are the small bumps found on the skin of those with acne.) That includes the 300 Kitavans who were between 15 and 25 years old. Not one person had a pimple. Among a similarly sized pool of adolescents in an industrialized society, 120 would be expected to demonstrate signs of acne.

And the same study reported similar results among the Aché hunter-gatherers of eastern Paraguay. In fact, the Aché results were even more impressive, because the researchers continued to visit the population over a period of more than two years. During that time, the number of active cases of acne they observed was zero.

———

That our contemporary industrialized lifestyle is affecting the skin is increasingly accepted among dermatologists. The authors of the above study focused on the effects of the industrialized *diet* on acne rates, speculating that both the Aché and Kitavan people ate mostly unprocessed foods—with few of the carbohydrates we tend to consume in contemporary society. Such carbs, researchers believe, cause high glycemic levels that could lead to long-term elevation of blood insulin, which has been linked to increased incidence of acne. Perhaps, researchers speculated, a diet of low-glycemic-index foods could lead to decreased levels of acne in industrialized societies. (Other researchers have since confirmed the hypothesis.)

In other words, a classic element of contemporary living—diet—was shown to affect the skin. But I think it's more than that: Another key component of industrialized living is changing the skin's ability to act as a barrier to the outside world.

That key component is the way we take care of our skin. I think we're washing too much. We're also using far too many skincare products. Daily washing of our babies and children is now thought to have contributed to the steep rise in cases of eczema, asthma and hay fever. And then, in adulthood, our incessant washing, moisturizing, exfoliating, cleansing and polishing—I think it's *damaging* the skin. The numerous actions we take every day to protect and care for our skin can actually end up doing the opposite. All the products we're using can instead compromise the skin's barrier function, damaging its ability to work the way it should.

Skin Basics: Nature's Most Sophisticated Membrane

To understand how overwashing and overfrequent product use may be damaging the skin, we need to understand how skin works. The body's largest organ has evolved over the course of millions of years to be one of the most sophisticated membranes nature ever invented. The skin functions as our body's armour, protecting our muscles and internal organs from things like sunlight, harmful germs and substances the body might find toxic. Skin insulates our internal organs from extremes of cold and heat, allows nerves to convey information to the brain about the external world and just in general works like the perfect permeable barrier—keeping good stuff like water in and bad stuff like toxins and allergens out.

The average adult human body features about 1.8 square metres of the stuff, although of course that amount varies with a person's size and shape. Elizabeth Grice and Julie Segre, of the National Human Genome Research Institute in Bethesda, Maryland, describe the skin as an "ecosystem," one that is "composed of living biological and physical components occupying diverse habitats."

Human skin is in fact a collection of different ecosystems, just like the world at large. Rather than jungle and desert and swamp, the skin has the scalp, which features lots of hair follicles and sebaceous glands, also known as oil glands. The underarm and groin tend to be dark, humid places, again with their share of hair follicles and sebaceous glands. And then the skin of the arms and legs tends to feature fewer hair follicles and relatively few sebaceous glands. The point? What's at your elbow doesn't look much like the stuff on your forehead—but it's skin just the same.

Skin actually consists of three layers. The deepest layer is the *hypodermis*, which includes fat tissue as well as larger blood vessels and nerves. It's also where you'll find the roots of hair follicles and some glands.

Closer to the surface is the *dermis*, which contains your collagen and elastin. Sweat glands live in the dermis—they emit moisture to cool the skin and the rest of the body. Although these glands are located across the human body, there are many more sweat glands on the soles of the feet, on the palms and on the head. And certain kinds of sweat glands, the apocrine glands located in the armpits and genital regions, are triggered by the presence of adrenalin. They emit a milky substance that may contain the pheromones that provide triggers to other people—said to attract genetically appropriate sexual partners. Also living in the dermis are oil glands, which secrete something called *sebum*. It lubricates the cells; it creates a fluid through which flow things that aid the health of the skin, like antioxidants; and it protects the body against harmful germs by forming a thin layer of acid on the skin surface. Known as the acid "mantle," this layer helps to regulate the number of bacteria and viruses that live on the skin.

Bear in mind that the thickness of the dermis differs in different parts of the body. Our dermis also thins with age—which is why many beauty products try to fight the appearance of aging by providing the dermis with additional collagen and elastin. No matter our age, the dermis is thinnest at the eyelids and thickest at the heel. One thing to remember about the dermis is that it doesn't regenerate. You only get one dermis. Say you break a glass one night when washing dishes. If the cut slices through to the dermis, you'll get a scar.

Now for the skin's outermost layer—the *epidermis*—which we'll spend the rest of the chapter discussing. On a microscopic level the epidermis functions a bit like a brick-and-mortar wall, protecting us from the outside world. This brick-and-mortar concept is one of the most important in the book. It's integral to understanding what overwashing is doing to our skin.

The bricks in our analogy are our skin cells, known as keratinocytes. The newest, living cells are produced at the deepest layers of the epidermis. As each successive layer is generated, it pushes the other layers out. The keratinocyte dies along the journey, and then once it nears the surface it flattens and hardens until, at the rate of about a layer a day, it sloughs off to be replaced by the next, newer layer underneath it. The whole process is a bit like a conveyor belt of skin cells. The outermost layer of the epidermis, known as the stratum corneum, has about 15 layers of keratinocytes and completely regenerates every two weeks or so. This conveyor-belt regeneration process is why, when you scrape your knee, the new skin grows back without any scar. Around 5 percent of the cells in the epidermis are things other than keratinocytes. Melanocytes produce the pigment, melanin, which gives us our skin colour and our ability to tan. Immune-system cells act as sentinels that warn the rest of the immune system of the presence in the skin of certain toxins or germs.

The mortar holding those bricks in place is lipids—fat molecules called ceramides or fatty acids. Together, the keratinocyte bricks and the lipid mortar form our skin barrier—our armour. And if the barrier is damaged, the skin cannot function properly. It can't protect what's underneath like it should, allowing potential pathogens, irritants and allergens to get in. Allowing moisture to get out. The result? A skin barrier that is not healthy.

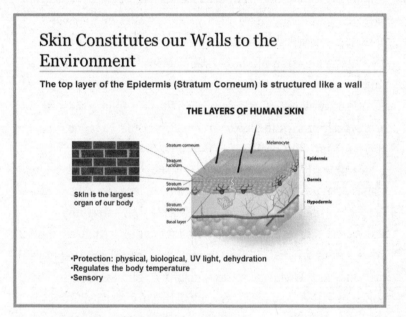

Skin Constitutes our Walls to the Environment

The top layer of the Epidermis (Stratum Corneum) is structured like a wall

THE LAYERS OF HUMAN SKIN

Skin is the largest organ of our body

Stratum corneum
Stratum lucidum
Stratum granulosum
Stratum spinosum
Basal layer
Melanocyte
Epidermis
Dermis
Hypodermis

•Protection: physical, biological, UV light, dehydration
•Regulates the body temperature
•Sensory

Source: Apostolos Pappas, PhD. Used with permission.

Sensitive Skin and Skin Health

So how does sensitive skin play into all this? First, let's define the condition. The medical profession hasn't come to a clinical consensus on that, but American dermatologist Howard Maibach, considered the leading authority on the topic, says in the book he co-edited, *Sensitive Skin Syndrome*, that the condition is characterized by "subjective cutaneous hyper-reactivity to environmental factors."

If we take the lab coat off those words and translate them for non-medical people, that mouthful means that the external environment causes the skin of sufferers to feel extra sensitive.

Sounds obvious, doesn't it?

Basically, if your skin frequently gets irritated from over-the-counter skincare products or even fabrics like wool, or if you just have itchy, burning skin frequently or intermittently, then you probably have sensitive skin.

But the more important question here is *why*. Why is this happening? Let's start by examining exactly what's going on.

Sensitive skin is most common on the face, followed by the hands, scalp and groin. In a few unlucky patients, I've seen the condition manifest itself across the entire body. The sensitivity can grow worse when sufferers wash, apply sunscreen or use cosmetics. Climate can play a factor: Dry air can worsen it, as can cold climates. In fact, I've seen everything from air conditioning to clothing to sunscreen bring on a bout of sensitive skin. And as Maibach himself notes, some patients don't experience *any* external manifestation of the condition. That is, sometimes there's no redness or rash. The only sign of the condition is the actual hypersensitivity. Other times, just to make things *more* confusing, the sensitive skin can get red, become dry or manifest a rash—or all three together.

In my clinical experience, two different pathways lead to the majority of sensitive-skin cases. The first is pre-existing skin conditions, and the second is something I call invisible irritation. There are other, rarer ways to get sensitive skin. For example, some people are sensitive to the sun or to climate, or they have a genetic condition that leads to sensitive skin. There's also something called immune hyper-reactivity, the causes of which are unknown at this time.

But approximately 80 percent of the sensitive-skin cases I see stem from pre-existing skin conditions and invisible irritation. And each one of those problems originates with a compromised barrier function. That's a problem that occurs when the outer layer of the skin—that brick wall of the epidermis—isn't as able to protect the skin's deeper layers from the external world to the extent that it should. The barrier has holes in it, allowing stuff to get in that shouldn't, causing a reaction.

The plain fact of the matter is that the majority of cases of sensitive skin have to do with the habits of modern society. The way we're supposedly "taking care" of our skin today ends up doing the opposite—damaging the skin's barrier function. That's why we have an increase in skin reactions in patients worldwide. Most of the cases of sensitive skin I see are caused by overwashing, overfrequent product use and the use of too many different products. That's what I encounter in my office every day. And when we address those root causes—when my patients wash less frequently, when they wash fewer places all over the body, when they use their products less frequently and use fewer products overall—then their skin problems tend to go away.

Pre-Existing Skin Conditions

The first pathway to sensitive skin, and the most common one, involves a pre-existing skin condition. These patients have some sort of visible manifestation of the problem. A rash or redness, maybe. Some sort of scaling or dryness.

For example, consider rosacea—a chronic condition that results in redness on the face where people tend to blush, such as the forehead, the cheeks and the tip of the nose. Many patients come to me frustrated because they've already been prescribed medication to treat their rosacea—and yet the condition isn't improving. That's usually because they're disrupting their skin barrier with overwashing and likely irritating the skin with product use. No amount of rosacea medication will work if you're constantly irritating the skin with various cleansers and other products.

Another condition that results in sensitive skin is seborrheic dermatitis, which is the fancy medical term for dandruff. Most commonly understood as a scalp problem, seborrheic dermatitis can also occur on the face, particularly around the nose and eyebrows.

Finally, the most interesting pathway to sensitive skin through a pre-existing skin condition is atopic eczema. Eczema starts with itchy skin; then comes a rash that can appear on the face, wrists, hands or backs of knees. The rash can look scaly and thickened. On lighter-skinned people it tends to be red; on darker-skinned people it can look white. Sometimes the rash can get crusty and ooze liquid. Eczema also commonly functions as the first sign of what's known as the "atopic march," a group of conditions that includes asthma and hay fever as well as food allergies.

The incidence of eczema has been climbing in the last 100 years, and in the final decades of the 20th century the rates skyrocketed. For example, in the United Kingdom, eczema rates *tripled* between 1977 and 2007. Similar increases happened in Canada and the U.S., as well as in developed societies around the world. Today, in many countries, 15 to 20 percent of children have eczema, and it affects up to 3 percent of adults. Why the increases? One of the most current theories speculates that overfrequent bathing and the use of harsh soaps during infancy alter the skin's barrier function and its pH. Such practices also alter its microbiome—the enormous number of bacteria and other microscopic creatures that live on, and in, us.

The Microbiome

We're accustomed to thinking of microbes in the context of disease. We've been taught to think, Get infected by *that* microbe, and you'll get sick. But in the last 20 years, the development of genome-sequencing technology—which analyzes the information encoded in the DNA of any living thing—has enabled us to learn that all sorts of microbes are living on and *in* us, all the time. Besides human cells, the body also hosts such creatures as bacteria and viruses. In fact, there are more bacteria in the body than there are human cells. Some estimate that our bacteria number in the trillions, which would mean more bacteria exist in the body than stars in the entire Milky Way. These bacteria assist with the body's functions in numerous ways. They help us digest our food, fight off foreign invaders and regulate our appetite. They may even help stabilize our moods, with research showing that a healthy microbiome plays a role in warding off depression.

Lots of research has been conducted on the microbes that exist in the digestive tract. Comparatively little research has been conducted on the skin microbiome. But we do know this: There are a lot of them. According to researchers, the skin can harbour up to one million microorganisms *per square centimetre*. And we're talking thousands of different kinds. A survey of bacteria on the palms of just 51 people found 4742 different species. Each individual palm hosted an average of 158 different species of microbe. And what constitutes the skin's microbiome changes depending on which part of the body you're examining. What's on the foot is different from what's on your scalp. What's on your right hand might be different from what's on your left. The darkest, warmest and most moist regions—between your toes, the armpit and the groin—tend to harbour more bacteria than dry regions exposed to the environment, like the forearm and the back of the hand.

The microbiota, we're learning, play an important role in the body's immune response. In all areas, the skin hosts a collection of good and bad microbes. The bad microbes can make us sick. The good microbes *prevent* us from getting sick, sometimes simply by virtue of their presence, which takes up space that otherwise could be occupied by bad microbes.

Remember those immune-system cells I mentioned that exist in the skin? They keep a figurative eye out for substances whose molecular patterns are associated with disease-causing microbes. Those immune cells have to draw a conclusion each time they encounter a substance. They don't just differentiate, say, between a friendly skin cell and a microbe. No, it seems they're also able to differentiate between *friendly* bacteria and *harmful* bacteria. Good creepy-crawlies and bad guys. And if those immune-system cells sense a potentially harmful microbe, they activate a process that releases antibiotic substances onto the skin.

Some bacteria can help this process. The good members of the skin microbiome act as soldiers in a military outpost. They're constantly fighting incursions from foreign invaders. For example, a species commonly found on human skin, *Staphylococcus epidermidis*, produces a substance that inhibits the growth of disease-causing bacteria. Such microorganisms can also emit fatty acids thought to play a role in preventing germs from staying on the skin, which in turn prevents infection.

Bacteria and Health

When I went to medical school, a lot of health care involved one overarching imperative: Prevent as many germs as possible from "infecting" the body. That's how the medical profession had operated for more than a century, ever since the development of germ theory. A vast swath of my health education amounted to strategic advice for an unending war against all microbiota. Killing as many germs as possible, as frequently as possible. "For the past 150 years, we've been literally trying to just kill bacteria," said Dr. Jack Gilbert, an environmental microbiologist, in the journal *Environmental Health Perspectives*. "There is now a multitude of evidence to suggest that this kill-all approach isn't working."

Of course, many good things resulted from these efforts to reduce human exposure to harmful microbiota and viruses. We developed antibiotics like penicillin and vaccines that bolstered the immune system's ability to fight off infection. Mortality rates dropped steeply. Rates of such infectious diseases as cholera, typhoid, TB and diphtheria declined. Human lifespan increased— all good things.

But then in the 1980s and 90s, something happened: The medical communities in industrialized countries noticed a steep rise in atopy, a condition in which the body's immune system reacts to things it shouldn't. The atopic diseases include eczema, where the reaction is to things that come into contact with the skin, and hay fever and asthma, where the reaction is to things that are inhaled, like pollen. Also related to atopy are some food allergies, where it's ingested substances that cause the reaction. As I said earlier in the chapter, the incidence of atopy has been skyrocketing in developed countries. Take hay fever, which was so rare in the early 20th century that doctors had a hard time finding cases to study. Today, hay fever affects between 10 and 30 percent of the population worldwide. In the U.S., the figure is between 12 and 18 percent. In Canada, it's between 20 and 25 percent of adults. What's up?

In 1989, a British epidemiology professor named David Strachan was studying the incidence rates of eczema, hay fever and asthma when he noticed something interesting. In a long-term survey of 17,414 British children followed over the course of 23 years, children with lots of siblings were much less likely to experience atopy than those who had few or no siblings. When Strachan published the results in the *British Medical Journal*, he speculated that infections in early childhood somehow prevent allergic diseases. "Over the past century declining family size, improvements in household amenities, and higher standards of personal cleanliness have reduced the opportunity for cross infection in young families," Strachan wrote. "This may have resulted in more widespread clinical expression of atopic disease."

What was transformational here was the notion that exposure to infection was *beneficial* to human health. The theory that resulted from Strachan's short article was called the Hygiene Hypothesis. In the nearly 30-odd years since the idea was first proposed, the theory has undergone some tweaking. It's now acknowledged that exposure to certain microbes—ones that have evolved comparatively recently in evolutionary terms and tend to require dense urban settings to thrive, such as measles, colds and flu viruses—doesn't benefit the immune system. (Which is why the most important hygiene practice, handwashing, remains a good idea.)

However, the body does benefit from exposure to microbes that are "old friends"—microorganisms we've evolved alongside for hundreds of thousands of years, ones that our ancestors encountered in the untreated water they drank or in the dirt outside or with the animals they raised. Our bodies grew accustomed to having these microbes around from a young age. Eventually, we came to depend on them. These so-called germs helped to regulate our immune system.

Today we don't encounter nearly so many microbes, in part because most of us live in urban rather than rural environments. Now that our water is treated, our infections cured with antibiotics, our nuclear families smaller, our food maintained in sanitary conditions and our habitat often concrete and steel rather than forested trees and meadows, we're not exposed to the old friends we once encountered in the world from the moment we were born—in what Professor Sally Bloomfield calls "the right kind of dirt."

The result? The mix of microbes that lives in and on the body isn't as diverse as it used to be. Studies link decreased microbial diversity to greater incidences of atopy, whether that's eczema, hay fever or asthma, as well as other chronic inflammatory conditions, such as type 1 diabetes, multiple sclerosis and inflammatory bowel disease. The problem seems to happen like this: Without the proper mix of microbes coexisting with the body, the immune system doesn't work properly. Things that shouldn't provoke an immune response end up triggering just that.

HOW ECZEMA IS SIMILAR TO ASTHMA

I use this comparison every day with patients because people tend to understand asthma better than they do eczema. The two conditions are related, and often, both can affect the same patient. Say an asthma sufferer enters a room where people have been smoking cigarettes. The person with asthma isn't allergic to the smoke; he or she can deal with a little bit of exposure. But breathing in *too many* smoke particles tends to irritate the lung lining, leading to an asthma attack. And since the lining of our respiratory airways is similar to the skin, the smoke-as-irritant situation is similar to that of eczema—but here, any number of things can be the irritant that sets off an attack. Too much washing. Too much exfoliating. Too much use of a product containing an irritant, like a fragrance.

Invisible Inflammation

I've talked about how the first pathway toward sensitive skin involves pre-existing skin conditions like rosacea, seborrheic dermatitis and atopic eczema. Now I want to describe the second pathway toward sensitive skin and poor skin health: invisible inflammation. And it's this pathway that I believe explains the epidemic of sensitive skin in people who *don't* have pre-existing skin conditions. My theory is that this one arises because we're washing too often, using too many different products and using those products too frequently. And together, these three factors may be altering the skin microbiome and compromising the skin's ability to act as a barrier.

To form the microbiome, bacteria start to colonize our skin immediately after birth. Imagine this colonization as a mass migration. The first migrants move onto the skin at birth, from the mother's vagina if the birth is vaginal or from the mother's skin if the birth is Caesarean. And that migration continues to happen as the infant ages. According to one Johnson & Johnson study, "Timely and proper establishment of a healthy skin microbiome has a pivotal role in denying access to transient, harmful, and potentially infectious microbes. . . . Microbial colonization of infant skin is expected to critically affect the development of the skin immune function and perhaps the maturation of other skin barrier functions, as well as the development of the systemic immune system." In fact, a 2015 study in *Immunity* out of the University of California, San Francisco, theorized that, soon after birth, there's a key period during which the body's immune system trains itself to coexist with the bacteria that form the skin microbiome.

So what does our industrialized lifestyle do to our skin micro-biome from infancy? When we lather our entire bodies in long, hot showers and baths on a daily basis, and then, once we're dry, slather ourselves in moisturizing cream—is that changing the skin's micro-biome? And if so, could that changed microbiome be responsible for the epidemic in sensitive skin and other skin maladies?

First, let's take a closer look at what's happening when we wash. The sort of soap you might find at your local pharmacy can range from actual, chemical soap to a synthetic detergent, to a combination of the two—a "combar." Each soap molecule has two very different ends. One side of the molecule is *lipophilic*, which means that it sticks easily to fatty substances. The lipophilic end bonds with grease that sits on the skin. The other end of a soap molecule is *hydrophilic*, which means that it sticks to water molecules. The hydrophilic end bonds with the water molecules we use to rinse our skin, and as those water molecules sluice off the skin, the soap molecule pulls what's at its lipophilic opposite end—the grease.

So what's the problem? The soap molecule's lipophilic end doesn't *just* bond with surface grease. It *also* bonds with the natural lipid molecules that form the mortar in the stratum corneum's brick wall. And when we rinse off the soap, both the surface grease *and* the skin's lipid molecules also rinse away. With the lipids gone, we leave holes in the brick-and-mortar wall of the stratum corneum— compromising the skin's barrier function. In fact, soap can wash the skin into a situation similar to genetic eczema.

And that could also compromise the skin's microbiome. Two of the world's experts in the skin's microbiome, the University of Pennsylvania's Elizabeth Grice and the National Human Genome Research Institute's Julie Segre, point out that a "delicate balance" exists between host and microorganisms. "Disruptions in the balance . . . can result in skin disorders or infections," they write. Furthermore, they point out that cleansing can change the relationship between the skin and the bacteria that reside on it.

What's happening is that people are giving themselves a kind of eczema through overwashing. Then they apply moisturizers and other products that can further irritate the skin. And for some of these people, the skin doesn't even appear irritated. I see patients all the time who have itchy scalps, itchy legs, even entire itchy *bodies*— and yet they don't have a rash, or any visible evidence at all of the problem. In these cases, the skin *looks* normal, but underneath, the accumulated irritation from the daily or more-than-daily washing has created a troublesome case of invisible inflammation—a form of sensitive skin.

That said, from a scientific perspective, the effect of consumer products on the skin's microbiome is an emerging field. Cosmetics, soaps, hygienic products and moisturizers, write Grice and Segre, "alter the conditions of the skin barrier but their effects on skin microbiota remain unclear."

We can, however, make some pretty good guesses about how everyday beauty products affect the skin's microbiome. Let's go back to what's likely the most common substance among them, the one most of us employ every day in the shower: soap and its cleansing variants.

Whereas the skin surface is slightly acidic, with a pH between 5 and 6, soap is alkaline, with a pH between 9 and 10. Soap's alkaline nature can disrupt the skin's natural acidity. Handwashing with plain soap for one to two minutes has been shown to increase skin pH from 0.6 to 1.8 units—an effect that can last anywhere from 45 minutes to two hours. In a U.S. Centers for Disease Control paper, Dr. Elaine Larson of Columbia University notes that "some soaps can be associated with long-standing changes in skin pH, reduction in fatty acids, and subsequent changes in resident flora"—i.e., changes to the microbiome.

"Soaps and detergents have been described as the most damaging of all substances routinely applied to skin," Larson continues. "Each time the skin is washed, it undergoes profound changes, most of them transient. However, among persons in occupations such as health care in which frequent handwashing is required, long-term changes in the skin can result in chronic damage. . . ."

Possibly among the most damaging of washing behaviours is the use of antibacterial soap. The environmental microbiologist Jack

Gilbert was the senior author of a 2016 paper in *Science* on the anti-bacterial agent triclosan, which he says was found in about 75 percent of American antibacterial liquid soaps. That's despite concerns, according to Gilbert, that "triclosan contributes to the development of antibiotic resistance and may adversely affect human health." He points out that "exposure to antimicrobial compounds can disrupt the community of microorganisms that colonize the human body." And changes in the microbiota, he says, have been linked to "a wide array of diseases and metabolic disorders."

Gilbert is one of the leaders in a new kind of thinking about the microbiome. It's no longer thought that all bacteria are harmful to human health; rather, some are helpful. And the helpful ones work in part by crowding out the harmful germs. So when we use antibacterial cleansers, we're wiping out the good as well as the bad bacteria—and may be helping the latter by allowing them to recolonize the skin.

A Delicate Balance

To definitively establish that daily washing and overfrequent product use have harmed the skin microbiome, and skin health overall, we'd need to conduct long-term experiments. One experiment, for example, might require one pool of subjects to avoid using soaps and detergents from birth. Such experiments would, of course, be difficult to carry out. However, we do have lots of circumstantial evidence that suggests daily all-over washing and overfrequent product use are affecting the microbiome.

Recently, a team from the University of California, San Diego, led by the microbiologist Pieter Dorrestein, conducted a remarkable series of studies on human skin. One study was intended to discover what human skin might have looked like *before* the development of contemporary lifestyles. Before daily showering and washing, basically. So they did something similar to those acne researchers at the beginning of the chapter: They studied populations that didn't follow industrialized lifestyles. In this case, they collected skin samples from people who belonged to remote tribes in Brazil and Tanzania. And when they analyzed the samples using a mass spectrometer, they found that these tribespeople had a wider range of bacteria living on them.

Another study conducted by Dorrestein and his team had an American man and woman undergo whole-body mass spectrometry—a form of high-tech scanning. The team hoped to avoid having the results skewed by beauty and cleansing products. So they asked their two subjects to stop doing anything to their skin for three days before the analysis. For three days, the subjects didn't shower. They didn't shampoo, apply moisturizer or use cosmetic products of any kind. Even so, when the team conducted the analysis, the largest single source of the molecules found on the skin was *not* skin cells, nor was it bacteria, fungus or virus. The single largest source of the molecules found on the skin surface was *residue from beauty and hygiene products*.

"This illustrates that our daily routines leave molecular traces on the skin that can be readily detected and are a significant component of the . . . chemical environment of the skin," the researchers write. "The data demonstrate that the human skin is not just made up of molecules derived from human or bacterial cells. The external environment, such as polymeric materials in plastics, as found in clothing, diet, and beauty products, contributes significantly to the skin's chemical composition."

What studies like this are beginning to get across is that our contemporary lifestyle has profoundly changed the skin's chemical makeup, and, in all likelihood, the skin microbiome.

Erika von Mutius, a German pediatrician and the head of the asthma and allergy research group at a Munich children's hospital, speculates that the skin microbiome helps to shape immune responses, affecting the development of atopy and other diseases. Many others agree. The studies here are in their infancy. One of the most interesting is the Human Microbiome Project—an attempt by the U.S. National Institutes of Health to survey human microbial communities.

Strengthening the case that the skin microbiome influences immune response is a 2012 study conducted in the Karelia area of northeastern Finland. In that study, researchers first analyzed the skin microbiota of teenagers. The same teenagers were then tested to determine how sensitive they were to various allergens. The researchers found an association between the diversity of a teenager's skin microbiome and the probability that the teenager would be allergic. "Healthy teenagers had a greater diversity . . . on their skin compared with sensitized (atopic) teenagers," writes one of the researchers, Tari Haahtela, who speaks of microbes as "a living interface between human body and the environment."

In a textbook edited by the noted immunobiologist Graham Rook, an essay written by American chemical engineer David Whitlock and U.K. systems biologist Martin Feelisch states perfectly what I think is going on. "We hypothesize that modern hygiene practices, in particular the custom of frequent baths or showers with abundant warm water and lavish use of shampoo and liquid soaps, have led to the efficient removal of skin bacteria, including those that were once an important part of the 'normal' commensal microflora of the skin."

When we look at diseased skin—in eczema as well as in psoriasis and other skin maladies—the microbiome *is* different. It's less diverse. Has constant washing early in a child's life somehow affected the skin microbiome, contributing to the development of atopy or other chronic inflammatory diseases?

It's hard to deny that, over millennia, nature has evolved a wonderful technology, perhaps the world's most sophisticated membrane, to protect us from the elements and potential toxins and to regulate our temperature and moisture levels. And that over the last 70 years or so we've *redesigned* that sophisticated surface. We've changed it with an at least daily use of soap. With the frequent slathering of moisturizers. With the application and removal of makeup. And don't even get me started on body washes and shampoos. Through such practices, among others, we've taken the membrane that nature provided—and altered it.

So have we improved on nature? Has our alteration over the last 70 years improved on more than two million years of evolution?

I don't think so.

"Many dermatologists continue to battle an overwashing epidemic," writes Lily Talakoub of Virginia's McLean Dermatology Center, in *Dermatology News*. "From bar soaps to antibacterial washes, dermatologists continue to educate patients that the extensive lather, the alkaline pH, and the antibacterial components of our washing rituals can strip the natural oils from the skin and leave it dry, cracked, and damaged."

Which in turn, in my opinion, often leads to, you guessed it—sensitive skin.

HOW TO THINK ABOUT MICROBES AND THE IMMUNE SYSTEM

Some time ago I came across a great analogy that makes the link between the microbiome and chronic inflammatory diseases much easier to understand. I found it in an academic paper written by a British team that specializes in the microbiome's implications for human health. The immune system, the analogy goes, is like a computer. Just before we're born, the immune system has all the hardware and software required to do its job—but very little data. The data—in the form of microorganisms—need to be supplied during the first years of life—through things like a vaginal birth, breast-feeding, exposure to green spaces and close contact with siblings and other people. Which data you get dictates how well the computer works. And exposure to an insufficient amount of data prevents the computer from working properly. "If these inputs are inadequate or inappropriate, the regulatory mechanisms of the immune system can fail," write co-authors Sally Bloomfield and Graham Rook, both noted experts in the field. "As a result, the system attacks not only harmful organisms which cause infections but also innocuous targets such as pollen, house dust and food allergens resulting in allergic diseases."

Returning the Skin to Its Natural State

I'm not the only one suggesting we should step back from washing so much and using so many beauty products. One of the best-known outliers is an American company, AOBiome, which manufactures and sells a host of products designed to encourage the cultivation on the skin of an ammonia-oxidizing bacteria called *N. eutropha*. Along with respected dermatologists, the company has conducted promising double-blind placebo controlled studies indicating that the bacteria provide a host of benefits. AOBiome believes that the bacteria once existed naturally on human skin, but that frequent washing has now eradicated it from most of us.

Co-founder David Whitlock, an MIT-trained chemical engineer who wrote one of the papers I cited earlier, happened upon the stuff after a friend drew his attention to the way perspiration-soaked horses liked to roll in the dirt after workouts. Determined to figure out why horses had evolved such a behaviour, Whitlock took samples of the dirt and analyzed them in his home laboratory. One of the bacteria he found, *N. eutropha*, digested ammonia, which meant it was able to metabolize some of the most irritating and noxious compounds found in human perspiration, such as ammonia and urea. And *N. eutropha*'s waste products were integral to maintaining the ongoing health of the skin's microbiome. For example, one waste product, nitrite, controls bad bacteria. Another, nitric oxide, is an antioxidant and anti-inflammatory. But according to AOBiome, many modern cleansing products are lethal to *N. eutropha*, including surfactant-containing soap.

That's why these bacteria no longer exist on the skin of people who follow an industrialized lifestyle. (Significantly, in 2015, the well-known New York University microbiologist, Dr. Maria Dominguez-Bello, found the bacteria on the skin of members of the indigenous Yanomami tribe in rural Venezuela, providing further evidence that the industrialized lifestyle affects the skin microbiome.)

Sensing an opportunity, Whitlock and a team of associates created AOBiome and a consumer-products subsidiary, Mother Dirt. Their first product was Mother Dirt AO+ Mist, a probiotic spray intended to help *N. eutropha* recolonize human skin; in other words, to nudge one's microbiome back toward the state that nature intended. "Within two weeks of use, the AO+ Mist improves the appearance of skin issues including sensitivity, blotchiness, roughness, oiliness, dryness, and odor by replacing essential bacteria lost by modern hygiene & lifestyles," goes the marketing. Whitlock uses the stuff. Because of the bacteria, he says he doesn't need to shower—and he hasn't in 13 years. (He does wash his hands.)

A journalist named Julia Scott participated in a research trial for the company, which required her to go a month without showering or shampooing. She developed a body odour that she described as somewhere between pungent marijuana and fresh-cut onions. She didn't like what happened to her hair, either—she said it grew really oily. The changes to her skin, though, went in the other direction. Slowly, as the *N. eutropha* bacteria colonized it, "my skin began to change for the better," Scott wrote in *The New York Times Magazine*. "It actually became softer and smoother, rather than dry and flaky, as though a sauna's worth of humidity had penetrated my winter-hardened shell." Prone to breakouts, Scott's complexion cleared. And, she wrote, "for the first time ever, my pores seemed to shrink."

Through Mother Dirt, AOBiome has created a shampoo, a face and body cleanser and a moisturizer designed to work in conjunction with AOBiome's mist. "Our mission is rethinking clean," Mother Dirt president Jasmina Aganovic told one reporter. "Our perception of clean has become confused with the word 'sterile.'"

My point exactly.

I recently spoke with AOBiome co-founder and head of therapeutics, Spiros Jamas, whose company is participating in a number of scientific studies with leading dermatologists that examine the relationship between the skin microbiome and human health. "The skincare industry has been affecting this very large organ that we hadn't known existed," Jamas said, meaning the skin microbiome. "Now we're appreciating the role that the microbiome plays in these different biochemical processes. These chemicals we're putting on our skin are potentially having a damaging effect."

One of the most interesting things Jamas told me about AOBiome is how they got into the business of selling the Mother Dirt skincare products in the first place. When they launched the AO+ Mist, many of their customers kept asking them the same question: "Can you suggest a soap that won't kill the ammonia-oxidizing bacteria?"

The company headed to pharmacies and cosmetic shops hoping to find one. "We thought we'd find a commercial soap or shampoo that was friendly to our bacteria," Jamas recalls. "So we bought hundreds of products. Products for babies. Products for all sorts of skin. None of them—the organic, the babies, the targeted products, it all had similar effects." Every single one of the products the company tested, Jamas said, was harmful to the ammonia-oxidizing bacteria. "We didn't intend to be in this business," he noted. "But we couldn't find a commercial product that didn't kill our bacteria."

I believe it.

Damaging What We're Trying to Protect

The non-industrialized cultures I mentioned at the beginning of the chapter provide a good indication of the state our skin would be in if we didn't overwash and use too many beauty products too frequently. You'll recall that when they examined the Aché and Kitavan people, researchers found an acne prevalence of near zero. I suspect sensitive skin would see a similarly low prevalence—and that, overall, dryness, redness, irritation and possibly skin disease would be much less prevalent than they are in today's industrialized societies.

Skin is not just our body's biggest organ. It's the gateway that separates outside from in. The skin is what defines us. Contains us. It's the surface we present to the world. And every day, we're nudging it away from the equilibrium it evolved to maintain. Daily showering with detergents and the application of moisturizers, makeup, shampoos and conditioners that stay on the skin surface for days—these practices need to be rethought. It's hard to break habits we've been taught. It's in our DNA to want to be clean. But we have to realize that contemporary beauty practices go too far. That soaping our entire body daily is likely damaging what we're trying to protect.

To sum up, there are two main pathways to sensitive skin. The first is associated with a pre-existing skin condition, such as rosacea, seborrheic dermatitis and atopic eczema. The second, a pathway I associate with invisible irritation, is linked to the disturbance of the skin's natural equilibrium, the disruption of the skin barrier and of the microbiome. Both pathways can be activated by the too-frequent use of harsh cleansers and other beauty products.

What should you do about *that*? Read on.

4

Getting Skeptical About Marketing

Have you ever wandered the beauty product aisles of your local pharmacy and wondered, Where on earth does all this stuff come from? It's the sort of thing I might have considered once.

The sheer number of products out there is pretty astounding. One bestselling beauty brand has 21 different varieties of shampoo alone, and that's on top of its conditioners, shaping gels, hairsprays and holding mousses. You might conceivably stand in an aisle and see nothing but this brand of shampoo. You could reach your arms up left and right and touch hair cleansers perfumed with white grapefruit and mosa mint, cucumber and green tea and argan oil; shampoos adulterated with vitamin E and cocoa butter; formulations created specifically for the needs of long hair, curly hair or coloured hair or for those who want stronger, bigger or shinier hair. In short, segmentation by product and purpose and fragrance has created a remarkably large beauty industry, with annual sales somewhere between $250 and $400 billion, depending on how you tally up the receipts.

I don't wonder about the companies behind these products any
longer. Because I've visited many of them. It's actually a pretty
common marketing practice for beauty companies to invite
dermatologists to come and tour their facilities. For example, in the
spring of 2017, I flew across the Atlantic to the south of France to
tour the world headquarters of Bioderma, a 50-year-old privately
owned French company with 2000 employees across the globe and,
in 2016, €390 million in sales.

Bioderma got its start in 1977 selling a pioneering line of gentler,
"no-detergent" shampoos for people with sensitive scalps. Today it
positions itself as selling skincare products with a scientific basis—
one of the company's marketing slogans is "biology at the service of
dermatology" (hence the name, Bioderma). Along with five other
dermatologists, I toured the factory and its laboratory and met
marketing reps, heads of sales and, most interestingly, the company's
head of research. She told us about the way the company tries to
follow a principle it calls bio-ecology, which entails observing the way
the skin works, what it does naturally, in the ideal, and then creating
products designed to restore damaged skin and strengthen the skin's
natural processes. Along with such competitors as La Roche-Posay
and Avène, Bioderma takes a minimalist approach, limiting the
ingredients in its products to help avoid triggering reactions.

That's in direct contrast to the more-is-more philosophy
implicitly espoused by some publicly traded global beauty
behemoths. The epitome of this philosophy lies in the fact that
some of them continue to print shampoo labels directing
consumers to "lather, rinse and repeat." It's bad enough that some
people shampoo their hair every time they shower. And then here's
the label on the shampoo bottle suggesting that they shampoo *twice*
each time? All that shampoo isn't just washing your hair. It's also
covering your neck and your back and everything else with the
dozens of ingredients that sluice down as you rinse. And that final

word, "repeat," may not only dry out your hair—it may also leave you more susceptible to skin reactions.

AN ENORMOUS BUSINESS

Beauty and skincare are dominated by global companies that own and operate numerous brands, selling everything from moisturizers and makeup to toothpaste and deodorant. Here are some of the biggest conglomerates, according to market research provider Euromonitor International, which has ranked them by their market share in the beauty and personal-care product sectors. (Because the companies operate many brands that have little to do with beauty or skincare, the revenues and market capitalization below do not correspond to their rankings. Also, note that while Euromonitor did provide the companies' comparative rankings, the market research provider did not provide the companies' revenue information.)

L'Oréal S.A.
Based: Paris
Market capitalization: US$98 billion
2016 revenue: US$30 billion (converted from €25.84 billion)
Brands: Lancôme, Garnier, The Body Shop, Urban Decay, Kiehl's

The Procter & Gamble Co.
Based: Cincinnati
Market capitalization: US$232 billion
2016 revenue: US$65 billion
Brands: Head & Shoulders, Olay, Herbal Essences, Pantene Pro-V

Unilever Group
Based: London
Market capitalization: US$172 billion
Brands: Axe, Dermalogica, Degree, Dove, Pears

Colgate-Palmolive Co.

Based: New York

Market capitalization: US$63 billion

Brands: Irish Spring, Softsoap, Speed Stick, Tom's of Maine

Coty Inc.

Based: New York

Market capitalization: US$15 billion

Brands: Clairol, Cover Girl, Philosophy, Rimmel

What I want to get across is that the beauty industry is a business. A business in which the players perform risk analyses all the time. They make decisions that require cost-benefit calculations. And in these calculations the possibility of harming a small group of consumers can be outweighed by the likelihood of greater sales to huge numbers of people. That's why we still see "lather, rinse, repeat," on shampoo bottles. Sure, the repeated application might cause some skin reactions. But it'll also lead to significantly greater sales.

Behemoths like Procter & Gamble, L'Oréal or Unilever are the global corporations behind some of the world's best-known brands. They're many times bigger than Bioderma. Unilever's personal-care products business, for example, which is just a subset of the overall company, registered sales of more than €20 billion in 2016, about 50 times Bioderma's annual sales.

You might think I dislike these enormous conglomerates. After all, I'm arguing that the daily, all-over-body application of these companies' soaps, cleansers, skin creams and other products can disrupt the skin microbiome and harm the skin's ability to act as a barrier. That too much cleaning and too many skincare products aren't good for the skin. Which contradicts these companies' advertising.

But actually, I have a complicated relationship with the beauty industry. It's not unusual for dermatologists within my subspecialty, contact dermatitis, to be hard on manufacturers of skincare brands because we know more than most about their ingredients and what they do.

"Why do you put allergens in your products?" dermatologists like me complain to the companies.

"Less than 1 percent of people are going to have a problem," they retort. "So what's the big deal?"

That 1 percent is a big deal *to me*. Dermatologists like me see the pain and discomfort caused by those allergens. Yet the companies are full of employees who harbour a deep-seated desire to create and sell products that make people happy. The problem is, the structure of the industry, and the principles of economics overall, get in the way. And I know this because I've worked with some of these companies. Take Procter & Gamble.

Years ago, P&G hired me to help them market their Tide Free & Gentle line of fragrance-free laundry detergent pods. I didn't go around telling people, "Hey, buy Tide, it's great!" Instead I talked about how I thought that, as a category, fragrance- and dye-free products were good for people to use. Which I completely believe. Because they're less allergenic, and less irritating to the skin.

Through that experience I developed a relationship with P&G's Canadian head of marketing. In 2016, knowing my interest in the ingredients that go into personal-care products and the way such products are developed, she invited me to a small symposium that P&G holds every year for dermatologists. Known as the Science Behind Symposium, the event enables dermatologists to learn about the company and its efforts to develop new products. In return, the company solicits opinions from the dermatologists on the state of the marketplace, how to improve existing brands and what new products the market could use.

I was one of 10 dermatologists who attended the 2016 symposium. The trip happened at a fascinating time for the beauty industry. Through the 1980s, 1990s and 2000s the industry grew to a remarkable size, in part because it pursued an aggressive strategy of horizontal segmentation—which, in turn, has helped bring about some of the same problems that I'm writing about in this book.

Horizontal segmentation is relatively new to this market. A hundred and fifty years ago, most people didn't think to buy a soap brand. Rather, they'd go to the general store and ask for soap, the commodity, and the sales clerk would head over to a massive block of unbranded soap and cut off the size of chunk they wanted. A *hundred* years ago, if they walked or took one of those newfangled automobiles to their local department store, they would have seen just a few different brands of soap—Lifebuoy, perhaps Sunlight, maybe Ivory.

Taking a brand and altering its fragrance or flavour to appeal to numerous different market niches is a business approach pioneered by an American market research guru named Howard Moskowitz. He's been written about in the past, most famously by Malcolm Gladwell. When you go to the beauty products section of your pharmacy, grocery store or favourite specialty retailer, Moskowitz is the reason why you see brands that feature dozens of products, each catering to a slightly different niche of consumer with his or her own idiosyncratic needs and preferences.

Moskowitz first thought of this approach back in the 1970s, after Pepsi hired him to figure out how much Aspartame, the artificial sweetener, to put in Diet Pepsi. Moskowitz suggested that Pepsi create not just one Diet Pepsi but several, each of which would be aimed at a different niche in the diet soft drink market—those who preferred sweeter soda pops would get one version, while those who liked their soft drinks fizzy but not too sweet would get another.

But no one bit on Moskowitz's idea until 1986, when Campbell's Soup hired him to figure out what to do about its Prego spaghetti sauce, which was getting killed in the marketplace by Ragu. Could Moskowitz conduct market research to create a better Prego? No, he replied. I'll do better than that—I'll make better *Pregos*, as in plural. He would make lots of different kinds of Prego sauces, each of which would be aimed at a slightly different niche in the market.

Prego followed his advice, starting at the end of the 80s with the launch of a new extra-chunky spaghetti sauce—and it was an enormous success. *That's* when people started listening to Moskowitz. The food manufacturers realized, to make a metaphor out of spaghetti sauce, that people didn't just like their sauce spicy or plain or chunky. Some people liked things one way, others another way, and producers could sell more of their products if they catered to the strong preferences of many different people.

That horizontal-segmentation approach does a lot to explain the growth of the beauty and personal-care products segments through the course of the 90s and the dawn of this millennium. Take the Olay brand, the pink lanolin-based moisturizer invented in 1952 by Graham Wulff, who had formerly worked as a chemist with Unilever. P&G bought Olay's corporate owner in 1985 and, over the years, conducted a textbook horizontal segmentation with the brand.

Today, Olay features dozens of varieties. I'd say the closest thing to its original product is the Olay Active Hydrating Cream. There's also Age Defying Anti-Wrinkle Night Cream, Active Hydrating Fluid Lotion, Minimizing Clean Toner and Age Defying Daily Renewal Cream. There's eye gel and lotion with sunscreen, firming cream, facial cleanser and even Olay-branded facial-hair removers. And that's not even getting to the Olay sub-brands, which include such names as Olay ProX, Olay Regenerist, Olay Total Effects and Olay Regenerist Luminous, each one having its own various

incarnations, such as eye restoration complexes, intensive wrinkle
protocols and antioxidant sunscreens.

As a result of all this horizontal segmentation, in 2013 Olay
became P&G's 13th billion-dollar brand. And the company has
used a similar playbook with many of the other brands it's invented or
acquired—which include Ivory Soap (launched in 1879), Tide (1946),
Crest (1955) and Head & Shoulders (1961). The company has bought
its share of brands, too, among them Pantene and Gillette.

What underpinned its strategy for decades was an intense push
for expansion. "Our business model relies on the continued growth
and success of existing brands and products, as well as the creation
of new products," the company says in its annual stock-market
filing. At its peak in 2014, P&G's 165 brands sold US$83.1 billion
worth of products a year. The company has more than 100,000
employees, and in late 2014 its share price maxed out its worth at
more than US$250 billion.

In a *Harvard Business Review* article about the company,
Scott Anthony, managing partner of the consulting firm Innosight,
wrote that P&G in those peak years wanted to increase its sales by
5 percent a year—which, with annual sales of around $80 billion,
translates into sales growth of $4 billion. To reach that goal, P&G
created inside itself a growth factory to generate ideas for
addressing the needs of existing markets or for creating new
markets altogether. They were constantly brainstorming with their
employees, and meeting with consumer experts like me, to hear
these ideas. They spent billions in research and development—
$2 billion in a single calendar year, more than Bioderma's entire
annual sales. P&G had years where it spent $400 million purely on
efforts to understand its consumers. And its competitors set
similarly aggressive growth targets.

The result of this drive for growth can be seen with something
like Febreze, launched as an odour-eating air-freshening product

in 1998. Nothing like it existed in the marketplace at the time. There were products that *masked* bad odours in rooms by spraying different smells on top of the bad ones. But there wasn't really a product sold expressly to *absorb* bad odours. Febreze arose thanks to P&G realizing the market potential of a chemical, hydroxypropyl beta-cyclodextrin, a molecule that looks like a ring. The ring trapped scent-creating hydrocarbons, neutralizing odour—an entirely new market segment. And since the product first began selling in the U.S., it's been spun off into everything from plug-in oils, scented discs and, the latest invention, car fresheners, yielding its corporate parent more than a half-billion dollars in annual sales.

With beauty products, the strategy involves expanding not only into new categories but also into new flavours or scents. Take Pantene, which P&G acquired in 1985. Today, Pantene has shampoos intended to reduce hair breakage, to detox hair, to care for curly hair, to create hair volume, to encourage natural looks. All told, a casual count at its U.S. website reveals that Pantene has at least 21 different collections, each of which has at least its own shampoo and conditioner products. And that's not even counting premium blends and more tailored products for stylists. From the original Pantene shampoo, P&G has created a brand powerhouse with dozens of different products.

THE GLOBAL MARKET

For decades, such Western markets as the United States, the United Kingdom and France dominated beauty and personal-care products, with companies expending enormous advertising budgets to attract their consumers. But today, the most important markets are shifting toward the developing world. According to market research provider Euromonitor International, the Asia Pacific region accounted for a third of all retail sales in beauty and personal care in 2016, thanks to the region's enormous, and comparatively youthful, populations. Below are the five international markets that grew fastest in the five-year period between 2011 and 2016, with the fastest growth first.

Argentina

Population: 44 million

GDP: US$546 billion

Iran

Population: 80 million

GDP: US$393 billion

Pakistan

Population: 193 million

GDP: US$284 billion

Belarus

Population: 9.5 million

GDP: US$47 billion

Indonesia

Population: 261 million

GDP: US$932 billion

The View from the Inside

So what's the problem?

I'll get to that. But first I want to talk about my trip to P&G. The purpose of the trip was to demonstrate to dermatologists like me the kind of effort that goes into creating the company's products. Such marketing plays an important role. Several years back, with growth lagging and the share price underperforming, the company began a refocusing strategy that shrank it from 170 brands to 65. As part of the strategy, P&G sold such beauty brands as Cover Girl and Clairol to Coty in a deal worth $12 billion. Even so, in 2016, P&G had 21 separate brands that were worth at least a billion dollars each, including such stalwarts as Herbal Essences, Head & Shoulders, Old Spice, Olay and SK-II.

P&G also wanted to show people like me that it continued to serve its customers, aim for growth and think about new product lines, just as it had since the company was founded in 1837. So in May of 2016 I travelled to Cincinnati, Ohio, where P&G is headquartered. Cincinnati's a nice city, prototypically American, with a lot of history. The office complex manages to feel both immense and inviting; it has the atmosphere of a university campus. They seemed to have about 20 buildings, although we visited only two.

The first highlight was a visit with the director of the P&G Heritage and Archives, Shane Meeker, whom the company describes as its "corporate storyteller." Meeker provided us with a tour of the archives. Seeing the original packaging for Ivory Soap underscored the fact that it's been around for 138 years. Later, department heads gave presentations about the various aspects of their businesses. We looked at the science behind shaving, and male grooming in general, since P&G owns Gillette. Baby care was a big topic. And the research facilities just blew me away.

One of the things I'm perpetually dealing with in my practice is reactions caused by shampoo, so I paid particular attention during the half day we spent in the hair-research facilities. (Yes, P&G has hair-research facilities.) The shampoo division apparently houses the world's biggest collection of human hair. Next came a talk on beauty and safety by P&G's director of scientific communications, Scott Heid, who ensures that the ingredients the company uses are safe for humans.

I perked up at that point. Among the dermatologists, I think I probably asked Heid the most questions. "Why do you use *this* chemical?" I asked. "Why don't you have *that* product?"

We talked a lot about allergic reactions to shampoo ingredients. I really pushed him on the fact that some of P&G's products still contain the preservative methylisothiazolinone (MI), which, if you continue reading to Chapter 5, you'll learn is responsible for an epidemic of allergic reactions. Heid pointed out that P&G follows the EU's regulations on MI, which are the world's most stringent and shouldn't render anyone allergic.

Sure, I said, but other manufacturers *don't* follow the EU regulations, which is *making* people allergic, and when they *do* get allergic they can't use P&G products without getting a reaction. It would be better if P&G didn't use MI at all, I said.

We also had an exchange about my bugaboo, fragrance. I pointed out that when P&G puts fragrance in its products, consumers don't know the precise substances that make up the fragrance. All the company says on the ingredient list is "fragrance"—and that could mean a blend of 20 or 30 different molecules. It makes it really difficult for consumers to know what products to avoid, I said.

Heid was understanding on that front. If any consumer wants to know whether a shampoo contains a given fragrance ingredient, that consumer can contact P&G and the company will disclose that information, he said. But as he framed it, the greater issue is that consumers *want* fragrance. And he's right. That's what the market research shows. Shouldn't P&G give consumers what they want?

Not necessarily, I said. Not when highly fragranced shampoos and other beauty products can create reactions in some people. "Consumers want and need fragrance-free options," I said. The company has somewhere around 13 different kinds of Pantene shampoo. Can't *one* of them be fragrance-free? Because shampoo doesn't just affect the scalp—it also rinses down the body and affects all the skin it rinses over. Plus, those chemicals go down the drain and get into the environment.

Heid seemed really receptive to my input. And in general, P&G's answers impressed me. (In January 2017, the company launched a website to provide information about the preservatives it uses. Later the same year, it committed to disclose online by 2020 "all fragrance ingredients down to 0.01 percent for its entire product portfolio in the U.S. and Canada.") One thing I realized again and again through the course of my trip to Cincinnati is that the chemists and other scientists who develop P&G's products really do think about how best to satisfy the marketplace's wants and needs.

Lather. Rinse. Repeat.

So P&G's research facilities are very impressive. What no one mentioned during this trip is that the money to pay for all the wonderful facilities came from consumers buying P&G products. Similar facilities exist all over the world at the headquarters of its competitors. At Unilever, which is based in Rotterdam and London. At L'Oréal, headquartered in a suburb of Paris.

Recall that beauty products are a US$400 billion industry. Global skincare makes up a quarter of the beauty market, with annual revenues of US$111 billion. Geoffrey Jones, the Harvard Business School professor who wrote *Beauty Imagined: A History of the Global Beauty Industry*, says it's one of the world's most profitable industrial sectors.

And it got that way in part through the magic of advertising. Before it executed its focusing strategy, Procter & Gamble was the world's largest single advertiser, spending a remarkable $9 billion a

year to convince people that they needed its products. Its
competitors also spend billions.

"While the scale of the industry is impressive, its existence also
raises many questions," writes Jones. "What are consumers really
buying when they buy a perfume, or face cream, or lipstick? Why
do consumers pay so much for products whose ingredients are well
known to represent only a small proportion of the retail price?"

The answer, of course, is advertising. Big corporations like
Unilever, L'Oréal and P&G are full of people who genuinely want
to help and satisfy consumers. But these men and women work for
corporations, and these corporations exist for another purpose: to
make money. The glamour of the beauty industry, with its models
peddling skin-firming moisturizers and its "Don't hate me because I'm
beautiful" advertising spots, sometimes makes us lose sight of the fact
that these products are created and sold by publicly traded companies
that need to satisfy their shareholders with every quarterly report.
And they're not spending billions of dollars a year on advertising and
R&D just because they have a deep-seated desire to reduce wrinkles
on the faces of the world. Their shareholders tolerate these expenses
because the strategy also happens to be smart business.

That's why millions of dollars in research funding pays for
academic studies designed to support the use of these companies'
products. That's why our social media feeds, TV shows and beauty
magazines are filled with advertising that plays to the insecurities of
men and women. Are the pores on my face too visible? My cheeks
too wrinkly? Are my hands too dry? Does my forehead look oily?
What about my hair? Remember the Irish Spring ads that featured
the cheerful man lathering himself all over his body with the highly
fragranced deodorant soap?

Doing that every day is terrible for your skin.

People think they need to shower daily, to lather themselves all
over with soap or some other cleanser each time they stand under

the water. They think they need to shampoo their hair daily, and condition it each time they do. They think they need to apply moisturizer several times a day, with different brands for the face, the body, the lips and the hands. While they use one cleanser for morning and another for night.

Such practices started from fear—fear of smelling bad. Fear of looking bad. Fear of not fitting in. A fear exploited by corporate advertising throughout the 20th century. These companies had so much at stake in perpetuating that fear that they created an entirely new class of entertainment—the "soap operas" that were expressly developed to serve as a vehicle for promoting various detergents to mid-20th-century housewives. At some point the activities became routine. People don't think about washing anymore. They just do it. And they won't stop until someone or something tells them to stop. Which happens to be one of the reasons I wrote this book.

What's the point?

This stuff is a business.

That's why you can find shampoos in dozens of different scents.

That's why, when you go to your local pharmacy, the moisturizer section stretches high up and far below, to the left and the right. The same thing goes for body washes and soaps. Makeup and makeup removers. More choice equals more products, which equals more ingredients and the possibility of more reactions. The consumers want it, the producers make it, the skin reacts to it and the dermatologists fix it.

It's a spiral.

According to a 2017 survey of 3,000 adult women by the online beauty retailer SkinStore, the average North American woman applies 16 different products to her face before she leaves the house in the morning. The retailer calculated the portion of the products used each day cost a total of about $8, with women in New York, Connecticut and West Virginia spending $11 a day—an amount that SkinStore calculated could add up to $300,000 through a lifetime. That's a remarkable amount to spend on skincare products and cosmetics alone.

Still, it sounds about right for some of the professional women I see in my practice. After all, a fast-growing section of the facial skincare products segment is expensive prestige products sold in specialty retailers. And men are getting in on the action. "The momentum of men in makeup is growing," reports *The Globe and Mail*. L'Oréal's U.K. managing director, Vismay Sharma, believes that in five to seven years we'll see makeup counters for men in department stores. "Between my generation and my son's," Sharma says, "the taboos are very different."

Which makes the personal-care products industry very happy.

———

Some years ago I attended a meeting of the American Contact Dermatitis Society. Maybe about 400 dermatologists who specialize in treating reactions caused by the stuff our skin touches gathered in a conference centre in Miami.

One component of the conference involved taking the pulse of the Society. The intention was to learn what the dermatologists were thinking about their profession, and how the whole task of caring for people's skin was going. We broke up into small groups, maybe eight to a circle, with a facilitator asking the questions and noting the responses. I happened to be in a group with the Society's president at the time.

"Where do you think we should steer things?" was the gist of one of the questions the facilitator asked.

I suggested that the beauty industry be regulated, at least in part by tightening the restrictions on its labelling so as to make the ingredient lists clearer. "We have to do *something* about these regulations," I said. "Labels like 'hypoallergenic' aren't helpful for patients."

A colleague said, "I admire your altruism, your desire to change things, but it'll never happen, Sandy. It's impossible."

I encounter this kind of thing all the time. At a dermatology advisory board, say. Those are meetings convened by a beauty or skincare company, or possibly a pharmaceutical company, to learn whether dermatologists have any ideas about the sorts of products the market could use. "Where's a hole in the product offerings?" an advisory board facilitator might ask. Or, "What do you think about the products we sell?"

One advisory board I remember was for a company that had noticed a gap in the market for psoriasis treatments. The meeting, which took place at a hotel conference room in downtown Toronto, attracted about a dozen dermatologists. After the welcomes and the thank-you-for-comings, the company convener began by noting that there weren't a lot of over-the-counter treatments for the skin condition that causes patches of red, scaly, itchy skin. Maybe this was an opportunity to offer a product that would help patients?

If someone *were* to invent a natural shampoo for psoriasis, the convener said, where do you think we should start? What sort of substances should be in it?

The dermatologists began weighing in, one by one, going around the table. Let's add this, let's add that. By the time my turn arrived, the shampoo would have had a couple dozen ingredients.

Everyone's putting in way too many ingredients, I protested. Conventional shampoos with many different ingredients tend to *irritate* those with psoriasis. Something created to treat psoriasis should *minimize* the number of ingredients. A shampoo for psoriasis is a great idea. But make it bland, and fragrance-free, so it doesn't irritate the scalp.

"Yeah," someone joked. "We could call it the Do-No-Harm Sandy Shampoo."

My fellow dermatologists poke fun at me sometimes. They think I'm a little naive. But say you lined up 10 dermatologists and asked them, Do patients wash too much? Lather up too much? Do people use too many products? Are shampoos and skin creams and many other products too fragranced?

All 10 of them would say yes.

We *know* this.

The *entire profession* knows this.

And yet, after the sorts of advisory groups where I hold up my hand and take my stand, the market researchers tend to go back to their corporate chemists and add their fragrances and other ingredients because they think consumers want it. I say, Make stuff that's fragrance-free, use fewer ingredients, don't use preservatives that are allergenic. And they nod and say, We'll take that under advisement. Meanwhile they're thinking to themselves, The public *likes* scent.

So the next chapter is all about educating consumers like you on the sorts of ingredients that cause the most skin problems. It's about irritant and allergic reactions, the differences between them and the ingredients most likely to cause them.

But before we get to that, I want to finish with three points to remember the next time you're standing in a pharmacy aisle and considering whether to buy yet another beauty product.

1. *Less is more.* Every new product you buy and use is another product that could come with more ingredients, more fragrances, more botanicals and more preservatives, each of which poses an incremental additional likelihood of causing you a reaction. So the next time you're in your pharmacy beauty aisle, remember the principle of less is more when it comes to skincare, and ask yourself—Do I really need this?

2. *Watch the product-ingredient lists of recently acquired companies.* Whoa, that's some wordy advice. But listen: There's a product

cycle in the personal-care industry. A little upstart competitor will spy an unoccupied niche in the market and generate some sales with an outsider brand that stands for consumer-focused products. And then a bigger, more corporate competitor swallows the niche brand and takes it mainstream. When that happens, the new company will often change the ingredient lists—without telling consumers. So when a small and respected personal-care products company gets purchased by a larger competitor, keep an eye on the ingredient lists and be wary of any new, problematic substances.

3. *Remember that this is a business.* The personal-care products companies tend to serve two masters: Wall Street and Main Street. They want to give Wall Street growing sales—*and* give Main Street age-defying, fully moisturized skin. But sometimes Main Street and Wall Street head in different directions. Behavioural economics shows that, within certain parameters, more choice equals more sales. So when you're paying attention to product marketing, try to stay skeptical.

WHAT DOES "COSMECEUTICAL" MEAN?

It's one of the more unwieldy terms used in the skincare products industry—as well as one of the fastest-growing product segments. "Cosmeceutical" was coined by Dr. Albert Kligman, the Pennsylvania dermatologist who pioneered the use of Retin-A as a treatment for acne. The term captures an idiosyncrasy of the skincare industry, where a gap exists between medical-grade drugs scientifically proven to treat skin conditions and the beauty therapies marketed by consumer-product companies. The products don't require the approval of drug regulators like the FDA or Health Canada, but nevertheless may have effects on the skin that rival those of a drug. "Cosmeceutical" now refers to any powerful therapy that may reduce wrinkles and otherwise protect against the appearance of aging.

Smoke for Your Skin: Problem Ingredients

How many potential allergens and irritants touch the skin each day? In 2011 the Environmental Working Group reported the results of a survey of more than 2300 people on the use of such personal-care products as cosmetics, moisturizers, shampoos and conditioners. According to the survey, the average adult uses nine products per day, and among those nine products are 126 different ingredients. The average *woman* uses 12 products, which contain 168 different ingredients. And 25 percent of women use more than 15 different products a day. That's a lot of potential allergens and irritants. And sometimes, these ingredients cause problems for the skin.

Take what happened with Sarah, the first of what would become a wave of patients I began seeing around 2013. A pretty woman, tall and blond, she worked as a teller at a bank. But lately she'd been having trouble at work: She couldn't concentrate because her skin was so itchy. It also prevented her from sleeping at night. A rash had developed all over her face, neck and upper body,

and she scratched all the time, sometimes so deeply and
strenuously that she drew blood.

She'd gone to see a local dermatologist, who said she had
severe dermatitis, which was pretty obvious, given that
dermatitis is a medical term for skin rash. The dermatologist had
put her on a medication called prednisone, which is designed to
relieve an allergic skin reaction. The rash subsided a bit, but then
once her prescription ran out the reaction returned, just as
seriously as before.

Desperate, Sarah found her way to me. She told me her skin
reaction was so bad she couldn't live with it anymore. It sounds
drastic, but she'd even considered suicide—something that comes
up in extreme cases more often than you might think.

I moved quickly to test Sarah to determine whether she was
reacting to any common allergens. And it turned out she was—to a
preservative, methylisothiazolinone, that these days is mainly used in
rinse-off personal-care products. The same substance created the
reaction that affected Jennifer, the woman I mentioned in Chapter 1.
"Rinse-off" personal-care products are things like shampoo and conditioner, which aren't designed to stay on the skin for any significant
length of time, as opposed to "leave-on" personal-care products,
which include things like moisturizers, sunscreens and makeup.

Referred to by its short form, MI, methylisothiazolinone would
become the trigger for one of the dermatology field's more serious
waves of allergen attacks. But problematic ingredients like MI have
emerged every couple of years as the personal-care products
industry grows.

Lots of these products have water in them. Left alone in a
bathroom's moist environment, they could go bad and develop
bacterial overgrowth, within weeks of manufacturing. So the
companies that make them tend to incorporate some sort of
preservative into the ingredient mix. For years, parabens were

among the most popular of these preservatives. But then consumers became concerned about parabens, wondering whether they may have cancer-causing properties.

Consequently, manufacturers looking to slap a "paraben-free" label on their products searched for other preservatives. MI became one of them, except that it had allergenic properties. So at first it was used with a related chemical, methylchloroisothiazolinone (MCI); the typical mix was three MCI molecules to one MI. Keeping the MI concentration low and reserving it for use in rinse-off products would leave the risk of allergy low. At least, that was the apparent thinking.

Then, for reasons that aren't clear, companies started to use MI more. It began cropping up in products in higher concentrations, and *without* its partner molecule, MCI. It also started to appear on the ingredient list of products that weren't simply rinse-off. According to *The New York Times*, the number of products containing MI more than doubled between 2007 and 2010, to about 2400. Colgate-Palmolive drew criticism for including MI in the ingredient list of a popular mouthwash, Colgate Total Lasting White. Kids started getting reactions after companies began using the preservative in baby wipes. The reactions generated a lot of press attention because their appearance was so alarming. Think about where baby wipes are used on kids—the face and the bum. It was disturbing to see a violent, poison ivy–like rash on the genitals and the skin around the lips.

Dermatologists like me began to see patients suffering from the widespread and significant rashes that affected Sarah. And at first, our allergy testing didn't pick up the problem because we were testing for *combinations* of MCI and MI rather than higher concentrations of only MI.

Once I realized that Sarah was allergic to MI, I taught her how to find the substance on products' ingredient lists. Her severe rash and itchiness started to resolve each day she avoided the trigger ingredient. It took weeks for her reaction to settle completely. But once it did, she began to regain her life.

Today, in contact dermatitis circles, we refer to the "MI epidemic." In fact, the American Contact Dermatitis Society, to which I belong, named MI its "allergen of the year" in 2013. Google MI today and you'll see numerous accounts of severe allergic reactions triggered by the preservative. One of the more disturbing accounts, from Consumer Reports' Consumerist blog, details the way MI caused a full-body reaction in an eight-year-old girl that was so bad, the doctor said, you "couldn't see her skin."

In 2016, the European Union, which tends to be the most aggressive in regulating personal-care product ingredients, banned the use of MI/MCI mix in leave-on products. In 2017 it also banned the use of MI alone in any products designed to stay on the skin, including wet wipes. However, MI continues to be allowed in rinse-off products like shower gels, body washes and shampoos, as long as its concentration remains below 0.01%.

The regulations are considerably more lax in North America. In the U.S. and Canada, many manufacturers of personal-care products have reduced the extent they use MI, but it continues to be found in low concentrations in a number of leave-on and rinse-off products, including laundry detergents—to which I've seen numerous reactions lately.

———

There was a time when people who struggled with allergies to substances commonly used in cosmetic ingredients had to navigate a bewildering number of different ingredient names—each of which referred to the same substance. Let's say you were allergic to diazolidinyl urea, a formaldehyde preservative used in skincare. Another name for the substance is Germall II. It could also have been called Germaben II. Having so many different names for the same thing made it really difficult for people to avoid substances that could trigger allergic reactions.

Then along came the standard dictated by the International Nomenclature of Cosmetic Ingredients (INCI). This system requires that ingredients be referred to by a single, standardized name. Established in the 1970s, the list of 16,000 ingredients is maintained by the Personal Care Products Council, and is used in such jurisdictions as the U.S., the European Union, China, Japan and, as of 2006, Canada. The idea is to make it simple for people to avoid the ingredients that are apt to cause allergic or irritant reactions. Most companies are consistent with the names, but it's not mandatory.

NOT ALL ALLERGIES ARE THE SAME

An allergic response sees the immune system reacting abnormally to a substance found in the environment. The substance that provokes the reaction is called an *allergen*. The reactions typically fall into three categories. *Ingested* allergies are reactions to food, or things that are consumed orally. *Inhaled* allergies are reactions to substances that enter the body through the respiratory system, such as the lungs, the nose and the windpipe. And *contact* allergies are reactions to things that touch or are otherwise applied to the skin and mucous membranes, the fancy medical term for lips, mouth and groin skin. In general, my patients come in believing that their skin rashes are caused by something they've eaten. Few people ever suspect that an ingredient in a personal-care product could be the reaction's trigger. Foods *can* provoke a skin reaction, but the reactions tend to be hives, typified by circular swollen and itchy red areas that come and go. If the reaction is scaly, weepy and red, and lasts for days or weeks, the trigger is likely contact in nature—that is, the trigger is likely something you've applied to your skin.

Read Product Labels Carefully

The following are the sorts of terms found on an increasing
number of skincare product labels these days. And yet, few of them
actually mean anything.

- dermatologist recommended
- for sensitive skin
- free and gentle
- hypoallergenic
- non-sensitizing
- ophthalmologist-tested
- safe for kids
- tear-free

One of the labels I dislike most is "hypoallergenic." Pretty much
anyone can slap a "hypoallergenic" label on a product without fear
of retribution from regulators—because there is no binding
definition of the term.

Many companies do try to make an honest effort to include
fewer allergenic substances in such products. They also make
mistakes. Some years back, a team of researchers surveyed products
sold by California retailers and marketed as being for sensitive skin.
Of the 187 products surveyed, 167 contained at least one contact
allergen. That's 89 percent. And 11 percent of them contained five
or more allergens.

The one term that carries some weight is "fragrance-free." If you
see that on a label, it's supposed to mean that the product doesn't
contain any ingredients considered a fragrance under the International
Nomenclature of Cosmetic Ingredients system. However, I've
noticed increasing instances where manufacturers have begun to
use a loophole. They call something fragrance-free but include an

odiferous botanical ingredient, such as lavender or calendula, orange or mint. Many of these botanical fragrances are potential allergens. Also bear in mind that "unscented" does not mean the same thing as "fragrance-free." Unscented products can contain fragranced ingredients.

I tell my patients to basically ignore most of the terms that marketers use to exploit the thriving market of people who believe they have sensitive skin. If you're looking for products that are less likely to cause a skin reaction, look for ones that are fragrance-free and have few to no botanicals. And bonus points if the product has fewer than 10 ingredients.

Allergy 101

Other problematic ingredients besides MI have come and gone. Remember that sunscreen ingredient, PABA (para-aminobenzoic acid)? A key ingredient in the first wave of sunscreens sold in the 1970s, PABA triggered so many allergic reactions that it's used in very few products today. And new problematic ingredients may be being developed as we speak.

Before we discuss which ingredients are most problematic, it's important to understand some fundamentals. Skin-reaction triggers are divided into two big categories—allergies and irritant reactions—and which one your reaction falls into will dictate how you treat it.

The one everyone thinks they know is allergy. In fact, when most people get a reaction, they think that's why. "I'm allergic to everything," people say in my clinic on a daily basis. Most of the patients who come in with a skin reaction aren't allergic to anything at all. Allergy is one of the most misunderstood medical concepts out there. The term is often misused to describe *every* kind of adverse reaction. Many food or drug reactions are the result of *intolerances*—not true allergies. The same goes for reactions to skincare ingredients. An upset stomach from an antibiotic or a stinging sensation from a new skin cream is not an allergic reaction.

Allergic reactions to beauty products turn out to be relatively uncommon. When they do happen, the medical term for the resulting rash is "allergic contact dermatitis," which can include redness, scaly patches and blisters. There's almost always a sensation of itchiness.

Here's what's happening behind the scenes: The trigger substance, which can be anything from an ingredient in a beauty product to a dye in the fabric you're wearing, wrongly activates the body's immune system. The biological response that is meant to fight harmful germs gets turned on by the trigger substance. The rash and the itching is the body attempting to combat the trigger. It's your body going into battle.

Becoming allergic to something is a process. To develop an allergy you have to be exposed to the substance more than once, and often repeat exposures are required. Many of the allergies I see in my practice develop after years of using the trigger substance without any problem at all. This surprises patients, but it happens all the time.

Up to 10 percent of people will react to a cosmetic product at some point, according to the American Academy of Dermatology. Another interesting statistic? At last count, the number of substances known to be able to cause an allergic skin reaction was up around 3000.

It's not clear what prompts the body to become allergic to something. As I discussed in Chapter 3, alterations to our microbiome may be playing a role. And once you become allergic, you're allergic for life. The reaction tends to be worse where the trigger has been applied to the skin—but the reaction can also spread to other parts of the body. That can sometimes make it tough to determine what provoked the reaction in the first place. Another complicating factor? The reaction may not appear until several hours or even days after using the product. Think of what happens after you touch poison ivy. The reaction doesn't occur immediately; rather, it comes on hours after the exposure, and can grow worse over time.

SKIN ALLERGY BASICS

1. Allergic reactions tend to happen after repeated exposure to a substance. The reaction never happens with the first exposure because the immune system must first become sensitized to the chemical.

2. Once you've been sensitized to a substance, you will always be allergic to it. Once allergic, always allergic. You can't be allergic some days and not others. If you find yourself reacting only sometimes to a substance, then you're likely not allergic to that substance.

3. It's possible to use a product for years, without incident, and then suddenly develop an allergy to it.

4. Even a small amount of allergen can trigger a reaction, and the resultant rash usually lasts several weeks.

5. With each new exposure the reactions can become stronger.

6. The reaction can spread beyond the exposure site.

7. A reaction need not happen immediately. Rather, it can take hours or even days to present.

The final thing to know about allergic reactions to chemicals that touch the skin is that they can be definitively diagnosed only by a specific procedure called patch testing. Screening for allergies to things you ingest or inhale is done with *prick* testing, which is a different, less-involved procedure that can be accomplished in one visit.

Patch testing, in contrast, is an enormous pain in the butt. Or, more accurately, the back, which is where the process takes place. First, it requires visiting a patch-test clinic. I run one in my private office and at my hospital clinic, but there aren't many patch-test clinics around, so getting an appointment can require a long wait time. The process begins with my nurse applying 70 chemicals or more in small patches to the skin of the back. Allergy testing is good only if you test the patient for their particular exposures. So which mix of patches you receive depends on what you do for a living as well as where you live. There's a standard mix for North America, a different one if you live in Korea, say, and another if you live in Finland. Similarly, there's a series of allergen patch tests for all sorts of occupations, such as hair-dressers, mechanics, health-care workers and dental workers. The idea is to expose the patient to the chemicals they experience in daily life. The patches are left on for up to 48 hours. After the two days are up, you return to have the patches removed and have the skin of your back assessed for the first time. A third clinic visit, for a delayed assessment, is scheduled four or five days after the first application of the panel, or mix.

Did I mention that you're not allowed to shower throughout the whole process?

Lots of people claim they're allergic to things. But frankly, the test to definitively determine whether you're allergic is inconvenient. So I'll spend a lot of time with my patients learning about their cases in the hope that they're not allergic at all. In the hope, actually, that their reaction was caused by a completely different type of trigger.

A JEDI HIGH COUNCIL FOR DERMATOLOGISTS

One of the research groups that protect consumers from allergens and irritants is the North American Contact Dermatitis Group, a kind of "Jedi High Council" of 13 dermatologists formed in the late 1960s in the U.S. The research group maintains a standard series of about 70 chemicals that can screen for common allergens. To ensure that this series represents the most up-to-date list of common allergens, the dermatologists meet annually to pool the patch-test data they've collected throughout the year. They discuss changes to chemical exposure in both the cosmetic and occupational sectors; they also track allergy trends. Based on this discussion, the NACDG may then tweak its standardized series of patch tests, adding a chemical patch test here. Their data serves as a cautionary reminder of the growing sensitization trend in North America—and in true Jedi form, they also train the next generation of contact dermatologists.

Irritant Reactions

If allergy to chemicals that touch the skin isn't common, what else is causing reactions to personal-care products? The answer is *irritation*—which happens to be responsible for the lion's share of sensitive-skin reactions.

So how does irritation differ from a true allergic reaction? In lots of different ways. The key difference is that, unlike with an allergic reaction, in an irritant reaction the specific immune system—the part of the immune system designed to eliminate pathogens—isn't involved in triggering the reaction. An irritation can happen upon first exposure. Reactions tend to be immediate, and in direct proportion to the amount of exposure. Get exposed to a little bit of the irritant and you get a little reaction. Get exposed to a lot of irritant, and you get a big reaction.

Here's the other thing with irritation: You may not react every time you're exposed to the triggering substance. Other factors tend to be important as well. Whether it's cold outside. Dry conditions may trigger some reactions. Humid conditions may trigger others.

Irritant reactions happen in certain parts of the body more frequently than others, usually where the skin is delicate because it's thin, such as the face, the eyelids and groin. Irritation decreases with age and is more common in women.

Finally, skin irritation is *cumulative*. That is, an irritant reaction is more likely to happen the more you're exposed to a substance, or multiple substances. One of the most frequent causes of irritant reactions is just plain soap and water. Something called "homemaker's eczema" is caused by repeated exposure to common household items like soaps, water and detergents.

Another big source of my irritant-reaction cases is the use of too many cosmetic products. Typically, these patients are female, and they're washing, moisturizing, buffing or scrubbing too much. Maybe the problem is all of the above. Each day, they damage the skin a tiny bit—and eventually, the damage adds up until, one day, there's a reaction. Not an *allergic* reaction, mind you. But a reaction all the same, featuring a similar amount of chapping, dryness and soreness.

Think of irritation and the skin like smoking and asthma, a comparison I drew earlier, in Chapter 3. If patients with asthma are exposed to smoke, their asthma gets worse. But they aren't *allergic* to the smoke; rather, the reaction depends on the *amount* of smoke they inhale. An errant waft of smoke from a candle typically won't set off an asthma attack. But standing downwind from a roaring campfire just might. Smoke is not an allergen—it's an irritant. The reaction, in this case the asthma attack, is dose dependent.

An attack of skin irritation behaves similarly. Except in the case of the skin, the trigger isn't smoke. Rather, it's any number of the things to which we expose the skin every day. Things like water, soap, some personal-care products, cold temperature, the sun, low humidity or even pollution. Mix several of these together, repeat over time and your skin reacts with redness and stinging. Some days the combination may not cause your skin to react. Other days it will.

Beauty products with ingredients that are irritants are like smoke for the skin. A little and you may be okay, too much and you could trip the threshold and react. Mix several together, the irritation accumulates and you just might get a reaction.

SKIN IRRITATION: SMOKE FOR YOUR SKIN

1. Irritation is *dose dependent*. The more you're exposed, the more severe the reaction.
2. Irritation is *cumulative*, typically requiring multiple exposures, or multiple chemicals acting together. However, unlike an allergic reaction, irritation can happen after a single exposure.
3. Irritation doesn't necessarily occur after every exposure. Some days you may be okay with the chemical. Other times, you'll get a reaction. It all depends on what else you did or put on that day.
4. An irritant reaction can happen immediately after exposure, and can go away quickly after the exposure ends.

The Allergy–Irritant Game

Why does it matter whether something is an allergy or an irritant reaction? It's important because the course of treatment is much different. If I suspect an allergic reaction, then I'll send the patient off for patch testing, which, as I mentioned, can be tedious and inconvenient. But if I suspect an irritant reaction, I'll direct the patient toward the product-elimination diet, detailed in Chapter 6, which can also be inconvenient, but in a different way.

Take Astrid as an example. This 12-year-old girl had developed redness and swelling on her cheeks while vacationing in the Caribbean. I conducted a short interview with her: Had she used sunscreen while on holidays? Yes, of course, Astrid said. Where had she applied it? All over, she said, motioning to her arms, shoulders, legs and back. It seemed likely that the trigger was the sunscreen she'd begun using on her vacation. But what sort of a reaction was this? Allergic or irritant?

Astrid's reaction was irritant. Most reactions to sunscreens are in fact irritant and not allergic. But the definitive factor in Astrid's case was the fact that she'd reacted in just one place—her face— and yet had applied the sunscreen on skin all over her body. It's impossible to be allergic on your face but not your body. Had Astrid been *allergic* to the sunscreen ingredient, she would have reacted everywhere she applied the cream. Instead, thanks to the heat and the extreme sun, repeated applications of the sunscreen on the sensitive skin of the face caused her to have an irritant reaction. A negative allergy patch test to sunscreens confirmed this.

What happened to my patient Kim is another example. As soon as she came in to see me I could see the problem. A severe rash covered Kim's eyelids, neck and ears. On the recommendation of her local dermatologist she'd stopped using any cosmetics or skincare products on her face. The dermatologist told her to switch to Cetaphil, a gentle, lipid-free cleanser, as well as a "gentle shampoo"—so Kim went out and bought a Dove Daily Moisture Shampoo. But the reactions continued.

Kim turned out to be allergic to a fragrance, which I verified with patch testing. The Cetaphil liquid cleanser didn't have fragrance. But the Dove shampoo did, which surprises many people because the brand promotes itself as "gentle." In fact, that shampoo contained both MI preservative and fragrance—and it was the shampoo rinsing down Kim's face and neck that was causing the reaction.

The Trigger List

Now for the problematic ingredients that most frequently cause allergic and irritant reactions. I'll start with the allergens and then finish up with the irritants.

Meanwhile, bear in mind that a lot of misinformation exists out there. Lots of online blogs incorrectly refer to every skin reaction as an "allergy." One blog I saw recently said that phenoxyethanol preservative was the leading cause of allergic reactions—which is entirely incorrect. Another natural skincare blog described MI as a formaldehyde-releasing preservative. It isn't at all! So be careful where you get your information.

My medical specialty is skin reactions. This is what I do for a living. Not only that—I allergy-test patients on a weekly basis, teach this topic at the University of Toronto and attend the meetings and conferences where the most cutting-edge research is presented. On top of my own personal experience, I'm drawing a lot of this information from data compiled by the North American Contact Dermatitis Group—that's the organization I mentioned earlier that pools their allergy-testing data to track new trends and novel allergenic substances.

Here, then, are the NACDG's most current top allergens typically found in skincare products.

Note: Due to the nature of the cosmetic industry, where ingredients and products are constantly in flux, I'll keep this list updated online at producteliminationdiet.com.

Top Allergenic Ingredients in Personal-Care Products

The top allergens in personal-care products that I'll discuss in detail include the following:

1. Fragrances
2. Preservatives
3. Hair dyes
4. Lanolin
5. Synthetic detergents
6. Botanicals
7. Nail cosmetics
8. Sunscreens

Fragrances

I have a signature scent—a French perfume, Tubéreuse by Maître Parfumeur et Gantier, that I've worn for about a decade now. I love it, as does my family, but I never wear it to work because some of my patients are sensitive to scents. Which is something I get. A while back I was travelling in Europe with friends when we went into a shopping mall. We made our way to the perfume counter and were trying on various scents when one of my friends sprayed on a particularly strong perfume. Immediately I developed a headache, which stuck with me for the rest of the day.

Fragrance can be both a blessing and a curse—particularly when it comes to beauty products. A great smell can create a blockbuster product that makes millions for the company that manufactures it. Think about the first thing you do when you consider buying a new product at a store: You look at the package, then dab a bit of it on the back of your hand—and take a whiff. Whether it's a moisturizer, eye cream, shampoo or cleanser, how you respond to that scent will influence whether you snap up the product or leave it on the shelf.

The problem is, the same smell that sells people on the product can also trigger skin reactions. In fact, fragrance is what keeps me in business. It's the single biggest source of skin reactions I see—the most common cause of both allergy *and* irritation of the skin.

Also known as perfume, fragrance is a complex, fascinating and ancient industry. It got its start millennia ago, when the first chemists extracted perfumes from plants by pressing or steaming the fragrant material, creating an essential oil. The person desiring to scent the air then burned the oil, which is how the word "perfume" came to be—in Latin, *per* means "through" and *fumus* means "smoke." Perfume means, literally, through smoke.

The stuff is big business. "A hair product that is inextricably linked to an enduring scent is something akin to the holy grail for beauty companies," notes the Paris-based writer Amy Verner.

Verner points out that the neurological region that deals with sensory information also happens to assist in storing notable memories. It's why the smell of Johnson & Johnson baby shampoo can evoke feelings of comfort and warmth for so many people—the scent evokes a memory of bathtime. It's the reason the smell of Pantene can evoke images of lockers and high school hallways, thanks to the young girls who dashed into homerooms with still-wet hair from their morning shower.

The trouble is that fragrance can be highly reactive. Some of those same molecules that tickle our olfactory senses also trigger reactions from the immune system. Oakmoss, for example, has been described as a "deep, raspy, dark smell that conjures up a primeval forest," which was why it was used as the base of such well-known scents as Drakkar Noir. But then in 2003 the trade group that oversees the perfume and scent industry, the International Fragrance Association, banned oakmoss because components of it were apt to trigger allergic skin reactions in a small percentage of those exposed to it. The removal of this particular fragrance rocked the perfume industry.

Estimates of the number of different fragrances used in the cosmetic and skincare industries vary. Some people say 3000. Others, 5000. The point is that there are a lot of them, and they're used in everything from the obvious, like deodorants, to the most innocuous of cosmetics.

HOW DERMATOLOGISTS DETECT FRAGRANCE ALLERGY

Pragmatically speaking, it's not possible for dermatologists to screen for allergies to every single one of the 3000 molecules considered to be fragrances by the International Nomenclature of Cosmetic Ingredients system. Instead, they screen with *mixes* of numerous different fragrances. Fragrance Mix 1, for example, screens against eight different common fragrance molecules, while Fragrance Mix 2 contains a series of different molecules. We also explicitly screen for a few other specific chemicals. This method will pick up about 85 percent of patients who are allergic to fragrance. According to the most recent round of pooled data from the NACDG, 11.9 percent of people tested turn out to be allergic to Fragrance Mix 1, and 5.7 percent to Fragrance Mix 2. The numbers continue to increase year after year.

And more fragrances are being developed all the time. Fragrance chemistry is growing more sophisticated—which increases problems for people who are reactive to the stuff. Scientists, in fact, now have the ability to design any odour they wish. With a technique known as "head space analysis," they simply capture the air molecules that exist around the source of the target fragrance, perhaps a flower or an animal musk. Analyzing the captured molecules and recreating them allows the scientists to replicate the scent in everything from moisturizers to scented candles.

Those scents last longer, too. Over the last several decades, the chemists who concoct fragrance molecules have improved the delivery technology. "Encapsulated fragrance systems" are now able to place some of these molecules inside "micro-capsules." Many products now contain both free and encapsulated fragrance molecules: The free molecules can be smelled immediately, while the encapsulated molecules wait to be liberated by some sort of trigger before they release a fresh burst of scent. So the scent of your conditioner, which once faded as your hair dried, now can be designed to last for days. Some laundry scents can be designed to last for *weeks*. And the capsules can release their contents with various triggers, among them friction, light, changes in temperature and the presence of sweat or other moisture. It's great for people who like to get a burst of menthol when they lick their lips long after the application of their balm. But it's a big problem for people who are sensitive to fragrance.

Another problem is that, as I said earlier, cosmetic and beauty products carrying an "unscented" label aren't actually free from fragrance. These products are supposed to have no smell to them—but they contain a fragrance intended to mask the chemical odour of the product. Only products that are described as "fragrance-free" or "without perfume" are supposed to have no fragrance at all. And yet even this labelling, which we as dermatologists used to think was helpful, has been called into question, given that some of these products still include odiferous botanicals or other fragrance molecules.

Here's one example of that happening. For years, one of my go-to lines of products for patients with sensitive skin was called Cliniderm, because it featured a great shampoo that contained no fragrance or botanical ingredients. Then in 2010, Cliniderm's parent company was bought by a bigger, billion-dollar global conglomerate, Sanofi. Sometime later I began seeing patients reacting to Cliniderm products.

"That's strange," I thought. "Cliniderm doesn't have any fragrance. These people shouldn't be reacting."

But then I thought to check the ingredient list. And it had changed. The company had begun adding lavender, lemon, lime, rosemary and orange. Maybe they thought, as many patients do, that these substances were fine in skin products because of their natural origins. The new ingredients added a scent to the shampoo, yet because they qualified as botanicals, they weren't considered fragrances. So while the shampoo had a scent that could cause reactions, it still technically qualified as fragrance-free.

Which shows just how powerful a selling tool fragrance can be. So powerful that a smart company like Sanofi would risk compromising the Cliniderm fragrance-free brand identity. Scent sells when it comes to shampoo—as well as many other personal-care products.

Now, knowing that fragrance can be a powerful allergen, let's say you start reading the ingredient lists on your personal-care products. The trouble is, many of these lists simply mention "fragrance" or "parfum" and don't get any more specific than that. That really complicates things for people who are sensitive to a certain fragrance. The single word, "fragrance," could encompass another 20 or 30 ingredients in your product. And who knows whether the specific fragrance to which you're allergic is in there? Consequently, many patients have to start with avoiding *all* fragrance and botanical products. Once the skin reaction has dissipated, they can work on reintroducing fragranced products into their beauty regimen. (More on this process in the next chapter.)

Companies have avoided becoming any more specific because scents are so proprietary. What gives TRESemmé 24 Hour Body Shampoo its distinctive scent? That's a closely guarded secret: Check the ingredient list and you'll see only "parfum." The brand is owned by Unilever, the global consumer-care conglomerate. A dermatologist like me can ask my Unilever representative a specific question. Let's say I have a patient who is reactive to a common fragrance allergen like linalool. She's begun getting a reaction, and one of the many products she uses is the TRESemmé shampoo. I could call up Unilever and ask them whether TRESemmé contains the fragrance molecule linalool. And they would tell me. But that's as specific as they'll get—they don't have to disclose TRESemmé's full formula. No companies do, because the formula is considered a trade secret.

That said, the fragrance regulations are improving in some jurisdictions—like Europe, which in turn is incrementally improving things in North America. In 2005, the EU drew up a list of the 26 fragrance molecules most likely to cause allergic reactions. All manufacturers of personal-care products sold in Europe were required to explicitly list any of these 26 fragrances if their concentration exceeded 0.001 percent in leave-on products, such as a moisturizer, and 0.01 percent in rinse-off products, such as a shampoo. Nothing similar exists in the U.S. or Canada, although some North American companies do follow the EU directive because they export their products overseas.

One final thing to note about these 26 most allergenic of fragrances. Let's say you're allergic to one of them—again, say linalool. If that allergen happens to be a component of a natural ingredient included in a given product, the manufacturer doesn't have to explicitly list it. For example, lavender essential oil, tea-tree oil and peppermint oil all contain linalool. Manufacturers can get away with simply listing the essential oil without explicitly mentioning the linalool the oil contains—even under the EU regulations. Thanks to that, it makes sense to try to educate yourself as much as possible about the various components of natural ingredients. Read on!

In Europe, the following ingredients cannot be hidden in an ingredient list by a term like "fragrance" or "parfum." Rather, because these are considered the possible cause of allergic reactions, manufacturers who use them must list each one separately, by name.

- Alpha isomethylionone
- Amyl cinnamal
- Amylcinnamyl alcohol
- Anisyl alcohol
- Benzyl alcohol
- Benzyl benzoate
- Benzyl cinnamate
- Benzyl salicylate
- Butylphenyl methylpropional (Lilial)
- Cinnamal
- Cinnamyl alcohol
- Citral
- Citronellol
- Coumarin
- Eugenol
- Evernia furfuracea (treemoss) extract
- Evernia prunastri (oakmoss) extract
- Farnesol
- Geraniol
- Hexyl cinnamal
- Hydroxycitronellal
- Hydroxyisohexyl 3-cyclohexene carboxaldehyde (Lyral), a scent reminiscent of lily of the valley
- Isoeugenol
- Limonene
- Linalool
- Methyl 2-octynoate

Note that the EU overhauled the list in 2015. Three fragrance molecules were outright banned from being used in cosmetics: Two were the chemical allergens in oakmoss, known as atranol and chloroatranol, and the third was hydroxyisohexyl 3-cyclohexene carboxaldehyde, known by its acronym, HICC, or the trade name, Lyral. On top of that, the EU has called for about 90 more fragrance molecules to be added to the ingredients that must be listed in product labelling. About a third of these new substances are natural extracts.

Many companies that sell their products around the world, such as Unilever and L'Oréal, have adopted the EU fragrance guidelines in their labelling. But it's a different story with some North American companies that don't sell overseas. In the U.S., cosmetic and beauty product companies can get away with just listing "fragrance" or "parfum" and not being any more specific than that.

The EU labelling restrictions aren't enforced in Canada, either. However, the federal government's environment commissioner recently released a report that called on the federal government to more closely screen cosmetic products. Why? Because when an ingredient list in Canada mentions "fragrance," "parfum," "aroma" or "flavour," the product may include chemicals that can prompt serious reactions. "Those catch-all terms can conceal a range of potentially hazardous chemicals and this information is not readily available to consumers," the commissioner said. In fact, Health Canada doesn't screen cosmetics sold in this country and "cannot assure consumers that these products comply with the Food and Drugs Act and are safe." Basically, as summed up by one politician, the Canadian government leaves it up to consumers. It's "buyer beware." The commissioner's report also recommended that Canada bring its regulations in line with the EU's. In response, Health Canada said it was reviewing its plan and may move to carry out the commissioner's recommendations.

To sum up, fragrance is the top allergenic ingredient in personal-care products, so it's worthwhile keeping the following in mind when considering what products to use as part of your washing and beauty regime.

- More than 3000 different fragrances are used in cosmetics and skincare products.
- They're present in most types of cosmetics, including perfumes, shampoos, conditioners, moisturizers, facial cosmetics and deodorants.
- The fragrance ingredients in cosmetics are the most common cause of skin reactions.
- Cosmetics labelled "unscented" aren't fragrance-free, since some unscented products may contain a fragrance to mask another chemical odour. Products should be labelled "fragrance-free" or "without perfume" to indicate that no fragrances have been used.
- Fragrance allergy is increasing.
- Many fragrance molecules are naturally derived and therefore can be present in botanical creams that are labelled "fragrance-free."
- Labelling that identifies a product as "fragrance-free" may not be strictly accurate, since manufacturers are allowed to use odiferous molecules if those molecules qualify as botanicals, such as lavender, calendula or rose.

Preservatives

The next most frequent cause of allergic skin reactions is preservatives, which are included in cosmetic and beauty products that contain water—which is to say, most of them. Preservatives like MI, discussed at the beginning of this chapter, are included in personal-care products to prevent that moisture content from breeding bacteria or fungus, or otherwise decomposing. Kind of gross, huh?

Preservatives may also be called biocides and disinfectants, and they've been in use since the 1930s. There are lots of different types of preservatives, and many of them are safe to use if the concentration is kept sufficiently low. But as the concentration increases, the rate of allergy tends to increase as well.

Allergy to preservatives shows up in my office more frequently in women than in men, likely because men tend to use fewer products than women. The reaction tends to be a rash in the area exposed to the chemical. The skin can look irritated. It can be red, oozing and blistered, or, alternatively, dry and itchy.

I think of preservatives as a necessary evil. Not using them would radically decrease the shelf life of cosmetic products, which would make them even more expensive than they already are. Without preservatives, we'd have to refrigerate our shampoos and conditioners, or replace them more frequently.

Here, then, are the classes of preservatives that have a high rate of allergy.

FORMALDEHYDE-RELEASING PRESERVATIVES

Many of us recall formaldehyde from high school biology class as the stuff that preserved the frogs meant for dissection. It's also been implicated as one of the many things that can cause cancer. The U.S. Department of Health and Human Services classified formaldehyde as a carcinogen in 2011, but did not include formaldehyde-releasing preservatives. Even so, many skincare manufacturers are starting to remove this group from their products. Most people aren't all that thrilled to find it in their cosmetic or beauty products, even before I tell them that formaldehyde-releasing preservatives can also be potent triggers of allergic reactions. Designed to slowly release formaldehyde to prevent the growth of bacteria in a cosmetic over

time, the substances come with the following names, as specified by
the INCI system.

- 2-Bromo-2-nitro-1,3-propanediol
- Diazolidinyl urea
- DMDM hydantoin
- Imidazolidinyl urea
- Quaternium-15
- Sodium hydroxymethylglycinate

ISOTHIAZOLINONES

If you read the beginning of this chapter, you already know about
methylisothiazolinone (MI or MIT), the allergen that triggered an
epidemic of reactions several years ago. That epidemic continues.
The use of MI is now being scaled back by many cosmetic and
beauty product companies. But other members of MI's chemical
family can also be allergenic.

- Benzisothiazolinone (in some laundry detergents)
- Methylchloroisothiazolinone
- Methylisothiazolinone

IODOPROPYNYL BUTYLCARBAMATE

Long used in certain paints and to preserve wood, iodopropynyl
butylcarbamate has more recently been included in such beauty
products as foundations, concealers, self-tanners, eye shadows and
mascaras, moisturizers and shaving creams. It's one of those
chemicals that are said to be safe when used in low
concentrations—although dermatologists are seeing it cause an
increasing number of allergic reactions. The other problem is that it
can be toxic if inhaled, so it should never be used in perfumes,
hairsprays or other products designed to be aerosolized.

METHYLDIBROMO GLUTARONITRILE (MDBGN)
AND PHENOXYETHANOL

Frequently known as MDBGN, methyldibromo glutaronitrile has been used since the 1980s. But in the 90s it triggered an epidemic of allergic reactions, particularly in people who suffered from eczema. Some dermatologists in the U.S. were seeing positive rates of 11.7 percent—which, remember, represents patient pools rather than the population at large. In 2005 the EU banned the use of MDBGN in leave-on products, like skin cream, and in 2007 banned its use in rinse-off products. Very few products left on the market still use this preservative. Phenoxyethanol is another preservative that is often tested with MDBGN, but phenoxyethanol rarely causes allergy.

LESS PROBLEMATIC PRESERVATIVES

This list of preservatives have low to no percentages of allergy and are not parabens.

- Benzoic acid
- Caprylyl glycol
- Glycerine
- Phenoxyethanol
- Potassium sorbate
- Sodium benzoate
- Sorbic acid

PARABENS

Used since the 1930s, parabens are a family of chemicals that are among the least allergenic of the preservatives in beauty products—and also the most common. Parabens are demonized not because of their tendency to be allergenic, but because some academics have speculated that their use could promote breast cancer in women and sterility in men. The mechanism of harm involves the way certain parabens are apt to bind to human estrogen receptors. Further study is needed but no clear linkage exists in either case.

Of the four different chemicals from the paraben family that tend to be used as preservatives, butylparaben and propylparaben are the most likely to bind to estrogen receptors. (Comparatively unlikely, and hence much less harmful, are methylparaben and ethylparaben.) The European Union banned butylparaben and propylparaben for certain uses, such as in leave-on products like diaper cream for kids under three, and reduced their allowed concentration in other products. Since the ban took effect, most companies have stopped using butyl and propylparabens.

Hair Dyes

After fragrances and preservatives, paraphenylenediamine (PPD), a chemical used as a permanent hair dye, is the third substance most likely to cause an allergic reaction. It lasts a long time in human hair and doesn't fade with shampooing. (It can also be used in temporary tattoos.) A PPD-dyeing process typically involves two steps—first you apply the PPD, and then you apply the developer—with the PPD tending to be allergenic in its undeveloped state. Most often the allergy presents as a rash on the top of the ears and the eyelids, but in serious cases, the skin of the scalp and the face can become red and swollen and the eyes can swell shut. PPD has also been known to cause anaphylaxis.

Note that PPD-free hair dyes do exist. So if you're allergic to PPD, look for dyes that contain a related chemical known as para-toluenediamine sulphate (PTDS). Just 25 percent of people allergic to PPD will react to PTDS. But read the ingredient list, since hair dyes categorized as natural may still contain PPD, which may be listed in various other forms. These other names for PPD include:

- 1,4-Benzenediamine
- 1,4-Phenylenediamine

- 4-Benzenediamine
- 4-Phenylenediamine
- Orsin, Rodol or Ursol
- para-Aminoaniline
- para-Aminobenzene
- PPD or PPDA
- p-Phenylenediamine
- Related chemicals: 3-Aminophenol and 4-Aminophenol

PPD-FREE HAIR DYES

- Goldwell Color Chic (permanent)
- Goldwell ReShade for Men (demipermanent)
- L'Oréal Paris Excellence To-Go 10-Minute Creme Colorant (demipermanent)
- Sanotint Light (demipermanent)
- Schwarzkopf Igora Royal (permanent)
- Wella Koleston Perfect (permanent dye)
- Wella Color Charm (demipermanent)

Lanolin

Lanolin, a fascinating byproduct of wool, was a key component in some of the first beauty products of the Industrial Age. Sheep use it to keep their coats waterproof; once the wool has been shorn from the sheep, the wool is boiled and cooled, allowing the wool fat, or wax, to rise to the surface. The wool of a single sheep can yield about a cup of the stuff. Lanolin is mostly made up of fatty acids and alcohols, but a comparatively small component is wool alcohol—and that's what can be allergenic.

Some manufacturers of lanolin-based beauty products have decreased the amount of wool alcohol they contain to reduce their products' allergenic properties. Lanolin tends to be used in moisturizers as well as sunscreens, lipsticks, diaper creams and some self-tanners, although it can pop up in all sorts of surprising places. So if you have an allergy to wool alcohol, read the ingredients, where it can also be listed under more obscure names, such as adeps lanae anhydrous, aloholes lanae, amerchol and anhydrous lanolin.

Synthetic Detergents

We tend to associate detergents with washing clothes and dishes, but some of the substances that go into them also show up in personal-care products. These substances are known as amidopropyl betaine cleansers, which are later-generation synthetic detergents ("syndets" for short) that are derived from natural ingredients.

The first generation of syndets were based on sulphates, which chemists first developed as a better alternative to regular soap. Sodium lauryl sulphate and other sulphates create more lather and sidestep the problem of soap scum. But they can be irritating to the skin—and I'll discuss sulphate-based syndets later in this chapter when I talk about the ingredients that create irritant-based reactions.

To improve on sulphates, the industry came up with amidopropyl betaine cleansers. Cocamidopropyl betaine (CAPB) is derived from coconut-oil fatty acids. There's also a newer variation, oleamidopropyl betaine.

The betaines tend to be included in hair shampoos and conditioners, where they battle static and boost lathering. They're being used in hairsprays, too, which is a concern—why would anyone think to look for a detergent in a hairspray? You can also find them in dishwashing detergents and laundry cleansers.

Allergy to this group is low—but it's important to know it exists. There's speculation that the reaction's trigger can often be contaminants, with names like amidoamine and 3-dimethylaminopropylamine, left over from the manufacturing process that created the betaine. Reactions tend to present as a scaly rash at the eyelids or corners of the eyes as well as around the ears and neck. Finally, bear in mind that allergic reactions to shampoo ingredients rarely affect the scalp—I'll discuss that more in Chapter 6.

AMIDOPROPYL BETAINE CLEANSERS

- Amidoamine
- Cocamidopropyl betaine (CAPB)
- Dimethylaminopropylamine
- Oleamidopropyl betaine

ALKYL GLUCOSIDES

Also gaining popularity as an alternative to sulphates is a family of naturally derived detergents known as alkyl glucosides—which the American Contact Dermatitis Society named the 2017 allergen of the year. Made mostly of palm or coconut oil, the alkyl glucosides have a lot of things going for them: They were first developed in the 1930s, so they're well-established in the marketplace; they tend to be gentle cleansers that don't cause many irritant reactions; and again, for those who prefer not to use synthetic-based products, they're naturally derived. They've been known to cause allergic reactions, however, and according to my colleagues in the North American Contact Dermatitis Group, the sensitization rate is climbing, affecting 1.9 percent of patients screened by the NACDG in the most recent time period.

- Coco glucoside
- Decyl glucoside
- Lauryl glucoside

The enormous category of natural ingredients known as "botanicals"
has been hot for years thanks to rising consumer demand for
naturally derived skincare products. Used in topical cosmetics for
everything from colouring agents to fragrances, botanicals also have
purported skin benefits, including anti-inflammatory and antioxidant
properties. The FDA defines a botanical product as "a finished,
labeled product that contains vegetable matter, which may include
plant materials, algae, macroscopic fungi, or combinations of these."
The most popular botanical products are essential oils.

But botanicals can trigger both allergic and irritant reactions.
(I'll concentrate on the allergic component here, and on the irritant
category later in the chapter.) Consider what happened with Evolution
of Smooth, better known as EOS, a New York City–based company
that some years ago rolled out a line of lip balms in unconventional
pod-shaped packaging in every colour of the rainbow. A big selling
point of the EOS lip balm was its ingredient list, which EOS claimed
was 95 percent organic. The company aspired to using only natural
ingredients. It didn't use petroleum jelly.

What the lip balm *did* contain was a number of products like
beeswax, tocopherol and linalool, which, despite being all-natural,
also happen to be allergenic—they're well known to
dermatologists. Following the balm's debut, reports began
circulating of young women whose mouths broke out in rashes
after using it. In what would eventually become a 2016 class-action
lawsuit, one plaintiff described the way, once she applied the
natural lip balm, her lips became "dry and coarse," leading her to
reapply *more* EOS balm. And repeat. The next day her lips had
severe blistering—a condition that ended up lasting 10 days.

In fact, lots of the ingredients that appear in many all-natural
beauty products can be problematic for the skin. According to the
NPD Group, a market research firm, sales of high-end facial

skincare products marketed with the "natural" label went up by more than 25 percent between 2013 and 2015. There's a perception that such products are superior *because* they're natural. More authentic. Companies slap wholesome-seeming adjectives like "organic" and "herbal" on their packaging. The impression is of some early-civilization shaman employing an early mortar and pestle to grind out a plant's secret substance that will provide the key to everlasting youth and beauty.

There's probably something to the natural-is-better approach *when it comes to food*. Forcing chickens and cows to grow many times faster than they're supposed to with growth hormones and employing chemicals to boost the bounty of everything from corn to apples likely do little for the taste of the food, spell bad things for the environment and may set us up for more obesity, among other problems.

NATURAL ISN'T BETTER!

"It's your shampoo that's causing the rash," I'll tell a patient. "But my shampoo can't be causing the rash," the patient protests. "It's organic—all-natural!"

First of all, words like "organic" and "natural" aren't regulated in many jurisdictions, particularly when it comes to cosmetics and personal-care products. (In Canada, the term "organic" means that a plant or other natural material is certified to be produced without pesticides. In terms of beauty products, the organic certification means the entire product is made from at least 95 percent organic ingredients.)

More to the point, natural products can be every bit as reactive as synthetic chemicals—and sometimes they're *worse*. Take Aveda's Smooth Infusion Shampoo. It includes fragrances like linalool, citronella and limonene, which, despite being all-natural, are all on the EU's list of terrible 26 fragrances most likely to cause skin reactions. The Aveda fragrance is also known to contain ylang ylang, one of the more common botanical allergens, which is on the second round of the EU fragrance restrictions.

Plenty of harmful things are natural. Poison ivy, arsenic, even anthrax—they're all natural. The concept has nothing to do with whether it's likely to cause a skin reaction.

Things are different when you're talking beauty products. Natural substances have been used in beauty products for millennia. Botanicals were likely among the first, with ancient Egyptians using the henna shrub to paint their nails and colour their hair. Botanicals can be added to beauty products for all sorts of reasons. Some botanicals are also fragrances; they're in a product because they smell nice. Others are believed to have anti-aging effects. Some fight oxidation. Others may confer a calming benefit. Sources can be everything from herbs to trees, flowers, fruits and vegetables—you name it.

The problem is that some of the most powerfully allergenic substances out there happen to be botanicals. The most common adverse reaction to botanicals is a rash. One Italian study found that botanicals had caused 6 percent of topical herbal-product users some sort of an adverse skin reaction. That figure can surprise people, who tend to have the false impression that everything that comes from the natural world is somehow better for us.

In 2016, *The Wall Street Journal* ran a story about the problems of using botanicals in skin products. The article included a great line—a quote from Bruce Brod, a clinical professor of dermatology at the University of Pennsylvania and a past president of the American Contact Dermatitis Society. "I tell patients, 'eat organic, don't necessarily put it on your skin,'" the dermatologist said.

I love that line. Incidentally, whereas the chemists who created the EOS lip balms chose not to include petroleum jelly in them, I think it's great for softening and soothing lips.

And with that in mind, here are some of the most allergenic of the botanicals currently being used in beauty products.

PROPOLIS

Commonly known as "bee glue," propolis is created by honeybees; and is the allergenic component of beeswax. The bees harvest tree sap and then chew it up, with the resulting mix of bee saliva and tree resin forming the propolis, which the bees use to repair honeycomb. Employed since ancient times as a folk remedy, propolis is said to have antibacterial, anti-inflammatory and antioxidant properties. "The list of applications of propolis and its extracts is nearly endless," one study notes; they include everything from wounds and burns to psoriasis, herpes and rheumatism. In terms of skincare and beauty products, propolis appears as an ingredient in the Burt's Bees and Beehive Botanicals product lines, among others, and in such products as face creams, lip balms, shampoos and toothpastes.

I think it's fascinating that a product that is nearly three times as allergenic as parabens is so prevalent in the organic skincare market.

COMPOSITAE PLANTS

"Compositae" is the name of a family of plants with flower heads that consist of multiple individual flowers; another name for the family is Asteraceae. Numbering 20,000 individual species, Compositae include everything from daisies to sunflowers, marigolds, echinacea, chamomile and dandelions. Many of these plants are included in natural skincare products and herbal remedies, particularly shampoos. The allergic skin reactions they create can be rendered more serious by sunlight. Some allergenic members of the Compositae family include:

- Arnica
- Chamomile
- Daisy
- Dandelion
- Feverfew
- Marigold
- Pyrethrum
- Ragweed
- Thistle
- and many more

YLANG-YLANG OIL

A component of the recognizable scent in Aveda products and common in cleansers, exfoliants and anti-wrinkle creams, ylang-ylang oil comes from the flowers of the Cananga odorata tree, found in Indonesia, the Philippines and Malaysia. The oil contains such allergens as isoeugenol, geraniol and linalool. Sensitivity to the oil can develop in people who frequently handle products containing ylang-ylang oil, such as hairdressers and manicurists.

Other botanicals that are potential allergens include the following:

- Bulgarian rose oil
- Clove oil
- Eucalyptus
- Feverfew plant, allergen parthenolide
- Jasminium officinale oil
- Lavender angustifolia oil
- Lemongrass oil

- Peppermint oil, allergens menthol, limonene, linalool, citronellol
- Rosemary oil
- Sandalwood oil
- Spearmint, allergen carvone
- Sweet bay laurel oil
- Tea-tree oil, allergen melaleuca alternifolia
- Vitamin E, allergen DL-α-tocopherol

Nail Cosmetics

Adorning the fingers with long, shapely nails exposes the surrounding skin as well as distant sites to several powerful allergens, the most common being tosylamide formaldehyde resin. The resin combines with something called nitrocellulose polymer to form the tough, strong and shiny enamel used to coat fingernails. (Sometimes in ingredient lists the "tosylamide" is replaced by "toluenesulphonamide"; the two words refer to the same substance.)

It's important to note that this allergy differs from a standard formaldehyde sensitivity, and that a reaction can occur to both wet and dry nail enamels. In people who are allergic, the result can be a nasty reaction in areas commonly touched by the fingertips, such as the eyelids, mouth, chin and sides and back of the neck. Allergic reactions can also occur to butyl acetate, a solvent used in nail products, and to methacrylate-based glue, which is used in fake nails. The newer, UV-cured nail polishes, known as "shellac," that use methacrylate acid esters that can create allergic reactions as well.

Sunscreens

Most sunscreens have four components. There's some sort of active chemical that blocks the sun's UV rays. There's a base, which helps deliver the active ingredients. Then there's a preservative, to prevent it from growing mould or bacteria, and some sort of fragrance to keep the whole thing smelling nice. The surprise here is that not a lot of people tend to be allergic to the active UV absorbent. But some people are, and the most common of the absorbents causing the allergy are the benzophenones, followed by avobenzone. When a reaction does occur, the resultant rash can happen anywhere on the body where the sunscreen has been applied. Which is kind of obvious. What *isn't* obvious is that sometimes the allergic reaction doesn't occur *everywhere* the sunscreen has been applied, but rather only in those places that have also been exposed to the sun.

- Avobenzone (Parsol 1789)
- Benzophenone-3
- Benzophenone-4

It's easy to self-administer an allergy test for a given sunscreen, particularly if you're about to go away on holiday and have a new product you're aiming to try out. In fact, you can do this with any beauty product. It's called a repeat open application test. To conduct one, simply apply the sunscreen to a small, dollar-coin-sized area of the skin (I like the inner elbow or the side of the neck). Repeat the application in the same spot for several days. If no redness or rash occurs after three to four days, you're unlikely to be allergic to the sunscreen. Enjoy your holiday!

Top Irritant Ingredients in Personal-Care Products

The top irritants in personal care products that I'll discuss in detail include the following:

1. Water
2. Soaps and detergents
3. Fragrances
4. Botanicals
5. Alcohol
6. Abrasive scrubs
7. Vitamin A derivatives and alpha hydroxy acid
8. Shampoos and conditioners

Water

Ask most people about what causes skin reactions and they'll mention things like parabens (which are comparatively benign as a cause of skin reaction). Comparatively few would ever mention water. And yet water amounts to my single biggest problem for skin health. How could it possibly be bad for the skin? Because it's the universal solvent. Few things in nature are better at dissolving more things, and among the things it dissolves are the fats in our skin's stratum corneum—the outer brick wall. We knew back in 1973 that prolonged water exposure was a direct cause of dermatitis. That's why I suggest limiting baths and showers to less than 10 to 15 minutes. Any more than that and the water actually dries out the skin. People whose occupations require them to work with their hands in water, such as dishwashers, bartenders, nurses, food workers and janitors, should use gloves to minimize exposing their skin to water for long periods. And bear in mind: The hotter the water, the worse the resultant irritation.

Water's partner as the other most-used ingredient in skincare is soap and detergent—which also happens to be the source of almost as many skin problems.

I get a couple of patients a week coming in to see me because they can't figure out what's happening to their skin. It's dry. There's a sensation that things are crawling all over it. Often it's itchy, too. Many of them have office jobs; all they're doing through the course of a day is sitting at their desks and then going home, eating dinner, going to bed. But during their daily showers they're lathering and scrubbing their entire bodies with soap—and all that water and soap removes precious fats from our skin barrier. Over time, the holes accumulate in the skin's outer layer. So it's this daily, all-over-the-body exposure to soap that's causing the lion's share of the sensitive-skin cases I see.

What's the answer? How to prevent soap from causing so many irritant reactions? Basically, the best strategy amounts to quitting washing so much. You don't wash your arms and legs unless they're dirty. "You mean only wash my *bits*?" one of my patients asked me, incredulous. "Yes!" I said. "You've got it!"

It's amazing to see the figurative light bulb go on over people's faces.

In Chapter 7, I'll get into exactly the way I think one should approach showering and the role of cleansing in beauty regimens. For now, I'll restrict my comments to a description of the different kinds of soaps and cleansers, and their respective abilities to irritate the skin.

What most people refer to as "soap" are substances that chemists and dermatologists group into three categories. First, true soaps result from the chemical combination of a fat and an alkali, yielding a substance with one end that's hydrophilic, or water-loving, and another end that's hydrophobic, which means it doesn't bond well with water. (I talked about this in Chapter 3.) It's the dual nature of the molecule that makes soap function as it does. The hydrophobic end bonds with dirt or grease, and the hydrophilic end allows the molecule to be rinsed away by water. Such "true" soaps tend to have a pH of somewhere between 9 and 10, which means they're pretty alkaline. They're great at removing dirt and grease, but they also strip out the lipid "mortar" of the stratum corneum, the skin's outermost layer.

Second, and on the other side of the continuum, are synthetic detergents, a term often abbreviated to "syndet," as I mentioned earlier. Most people would refer to these products as soaps, but dermatologists and other health or beauty-industry professionals know that syndet bars include less than 10 percent of true soap. As such, they're much milder than true soaps. Their pH is neutral or even slightly acid, which is important because our surface bacteria require a slightly acidic skin surface. Syndet bars are less likely to strip out the skin's lipid matrix, but the problem is that they also may be less likely to remove grease and dirt from the skin. Also referred to as beauty bars, they include products like Dove, Cetaphil, Oil of Olay, CeraVe and Aveeno bars.

Third, and somewhere between syndets and true soaps, are what are known as "combars,"; these include products like Dial, Irish Spring and Coast. Combars "combine" alkaline soaps with syndets to create a bar designed to clean the hands and skin better while minimizing the lipid-stripping damage to the skin. While syndet bars are 10 percent true soap, combars tend to have more like 50 percent soap—which makes them that much more likely to irritate the skin with repeated, habitual use. They may also include an antibacterial ingredient. Combars are often what my older male patients will tell me they use. Take Alex, a 50-year-old businessman who plays squash three mornings a week. His post-squash shower sees him lather his entire body in Irish Spring soap, just like the television commercials. He also showers before bed—another all-over body soaping. Not surprisingly, he came in to see me complaining of skin dryness and the persistent sensation that his skin is crawling. I suggested that he switch from Irish Spring to CeraVe bar, and that he limit his washing to the genitals and the underarms. Voilà, his hypersensitive, crawling skin condition disappeared.

What about liquid soaps and cleansers? Liquid soaps mostly feature various types of synthetic surfactants. Surfactants work the same way as true soap, but they're made differently, without using lye, leaving them pH balanced and gentler on the skin. The most common synthetic surfactants used in personal-care products like body washes and shampoos are sulphates, such as sodium laureth sulphate (SLS), a contraction of sodium lauryl ether sulphate. While they create a lot of lather and effectively wash dirt and grease from the body, they also tend to dry out the skin, causing irritation.

However, as long as the sulphate concentration is kept low and the product avoids allergenic ingredients, I do prefer sulphate-containing liquid soaps and cleansers to natural soap. One nice thing about the sulphates? They tend not to be allergenic. Oddly, the alternative to sulphates, the betaine cleansers I discussed in the allergy section of this chapter, are less irritating—but more allergenic.

In Chapter 3 I described the way soaps and cleansers can irritate the skin. To sum up: The use of any but the most gentle of soaps and cleansers risks stripping out the lipids that form the mortar in our skin's brick-and-mortar wall. The same washing repeated over time is also likely to have long-term consequences on the skin microbiome. The result is small gaps in the skin's protective layer. These gaps allow skin moisture to escape and pathogens and irritants to invade the skin. The compromised barrier leads to micro-irritations that accumulate over days, weeks and months, leading some people to develop dry, cracked skin and, eventually, a skin reaction.

Fragrances

I talked a lot about fragrances in the skin allergen section. But they can also act as big irritants for people who are already set up for skin sensitivity, such as those who've created problems for themselves with too much water exposure or by overfrequent washing. Those who suffer from eczema, rosacea and dermatitis can be susceptible to fragrance-caused irritation as well.

The problem, as I mentioned earlier, is that consumers *want* fragrance. Fragrance in skincare is like sugar in food. We love the sensation. We want it—we almost crave it. But it's not good for us. Over time, fragrance use can not only irritate the skin, but also possibly lead to allergy.

Plenty of people can use fragranced products all they like. But others, despite not having an actual allergy to fragrance, may be susceptible to fragrance-caused skin irritation. One young woman I saw recently had suddenly developed a classic case. She'd suffered from genetic eczema most of her life, but over time had learned to control it. Except that lately her skin had been developing terrible rashes on her upper trunk and limbs— and the usual places where she developed eczema were also flaring up. Her family doctor was concerned that she was allergic to something.

I sat her down and we went through the sort of products she'd been using. "I don't use fragrance," she told me. "Because I know it makes my eczema worse. I only use natural products that are hypoallergenic, for people with sensitive skin."

To her credit, the young woman had been using beauty products labelled "fragrance-free." I've talked about how labels like "natural" and "for sensitive skin" mean very little. Still, patients tell me they want their beauty products to be more natural, and I get that. Some natural ingredients are great—just as many synthetic ingredients are. What patients should understand is that it's not black and white. No category is exclusively bad or good. Some natural ingredients are terrible for reactive skin. Favouring natural ingredients *because* you have reactive skin is not a rational strategy. I've said it before: Some natural substances are among the most irritating ingredients out there.

So let's get back to my patient. She'd done well to attempt to avoid fragrance in her beauty products, but she'd forgotten about the fragranced ingredients in her laundry detergent and fabric softener. That was the source of the flare-up. A university student, she'd recently moved away from home. Her parents had known to use fragrance-free laundry detergent and fabric softener when doing her laundry. But now that she'd begun buying her own laundry supplies, she was washing her clothes with the regular products—and the fragrance in her clothing and bedding was irritating her already reactive eczema-afflicted skin. Once she changed her laundry products to fragrance-free varieties, her skin calmed down.

Botanicals

Many botanicals are allergens—I discussed that earlier in the chapter. But the bigger problem with botanicals is the way they can also provoke irritant reactions. It drives me crazy. The skincare companies are marketing this all-natural and organic stuff full of botanicals to people with sensitive skin—when those are the exact people who should be avoiding these products!

The phenomenon is similar to what happens with fragrances. Water, soap, maybe some pre-existing condition like psoriasis—these can disturb the skin's barrier function, allowing something, in this case a botanical, to get past the skin's outer layer and provoke an irritant reaction: itching and rashy skin.

What applies to allergens also applies to irritants: The fact that a substance is natural has no bearing on whether it will irritate the skin. Botanicals are used in plenty of products that are marketed as "natural" and geared to those with sensitive or otherwise reactive skin. The trouble is that plenty of these products set their users up for an irritant reaction purely *because* of the botanicals. Recently, for example, I've been noticing that patients with fragrance sensitivities are coming in with reactions, typically a rash of some kind.

What's the cause?

The fragrance-free products they're using. Such products don't have any of the 3000 ingredients that are considered "fragrances." Nevertheless, they do have a scent added in the form of a fragrant *botanical* substance like lavender, lemon, lime, orange or many others. As I've said, it's a bit of a loophole—manufacturers can sneak fragrance into supposedly fragrance-free products by scenting them with botanicals. So for those with reactive skin, a more useful label would be "fragrance- and botanical-free."

Rather than a rash, some botanicals can make the skin sensitive to the sun, prompting the skin to burn a lot more quickly than it otherwise might. Coumarin, lemon, lime, grapefruit and bergamot are all botanicals that can make the skin photosensitive. Try to avoid the sun when using any creams, oils or hair products that contain these ingredients.

Public perception of natural-marketed skincare products was at the centre of an interesting case I saw recently. A mother had brought in a toddler with a terrible red rash all over his body. The boy had suffered from eczema all his young life. To help soothe his skin, the mother had begun using an all-natural moisturizer intended specially for young people, Abundance Naturally Baby Balm, which is marketed as a "therapeutic blend of essential oils and botanical herbs."

As cut-and-pasted from the company's own website, here are the balm's key ingredients, along with the company's explanation of why each ingredient is included:

- Calendula: Reduces inflammation, protects & soothes irritated skin and kills bacteria
- Chickweed: An external remedy to ease itchy, red, irritated skin
- Goldenseal: Contains natural antibiotics that fight inflammation
- Lavender: Reputed to heal burns, skin infections and sun damage

- Marshmallow root: Cools and moisturizes wounded inflamed tissue
- Sandalwood: A fragrant essential oil commonly used to moisturize

The crazy thing about this is that some of the above ingredients will irritate already irritated skin—in particular, the sandalwood. (On top of that, the lavender, sandalwood and calendula are potentially allergenic.) For children without significant eczema, a balm like this might be okay. But the people who go for this all-natural stuff tend to be those who already have reactive skin—and for them, I'd suggest they avoid it. Plenty of dermatologists have said it: All-natural is good for food but not necessarily for the skin. As soon as the mother stopped using the balm on the boy, the eczema calmed down.

Not all botanicals trigger skin reactions. Some botanical oils are very useful in skincare. Medicine is rooted in plants, and many of our modern-day drugs come from nature. What troubles me is when manufacturers throw botanical ingredients by the dozen into personal-care products with little science to back them up, and with most patients assuming they're harmless. Some botanicals are as irritating as almost anything else out there. So which botanicals trigger the most irritation? Here's a partial list. And bear in mind that new botanical ingredients are coming on the market all the time. This list is nowhere near exhaustive.

- Balsam
- Bergamot
- Camphor
- Cassia
- Cinnamon
- Citrus juice and oils
- Clove
- Clove blossom

- Coumarins
- Eucalyptus
- Eugenol and isoeugenol
- Fennel
- Fir needle
- Fragrant flower oils, such as narcissi, neroli and others
- Geranium
- Ginger
- Lavender
- Lemon
- Lemon balm
- Lemongrass
- Lemon verbena
- Lime
- Menthol
- Oak bark
- Orange
- Oregano
- Peppermint in any form, mint
- Rose oil
- Sage
- Sandalwood
- Tea tree
- Thyme
- Ylang ylang

ESSENTIAL OILS

Many essential oils can be irritating to the skin. Considered a kind of botanical, they amount to a blend of natural chemicals that have been distilled from the plant, often using steam. Some can contain more than 100 different chemical components. They're an attempt to create the "essence" of the plant—the substances that provide the distinctive fragrance or flavour of that particular species of flora. They're also used by some practitioners of alternative medicines. But according to the George Washington University Medical Center's National Capital Poison Center, "Many people think essential oils are harmless because they are natural and have been used for a long time." That's not true, as the Center goes on to point out—some essential oils are poisonous when eaten. They can also cause serious skin reactions. Moreover, children may be more susceptible to skin reactions triggered by essential oils. So rather than accepting essential oils as a natural ingredient, be cautious when using products that employ them.

Alcohol

Like water, alcohol is a solvent that can remove fats and oils from the skin—which means that it promotes the evaporation of skin moisture and leaves skin more susceptible to reaction from irritants. Many different types of alcohols are used in skincare, but because the concentration tends to be low, the alcohol in most creams or lotions shouldn't pose a problem for most people. Problems can arise from obsessive use of alcohol-based hand sanitizers—although proper use of such sanitizers tends to be less irritating to the skin than washing with soap and water.

Abrasive Scrubs

My patients frequently ask me whether they should exfoliate. Typically I tell them that the skin's top layer, the stratum corneum, renews itself every 15 days, so exfoliation isn't necessary—the skin's exfoliating itself all the time. But the technique does produce smoother skin. Also, the skin's natural exfoliation slows down as one ages, so some exfoliation from your forties onward is not a bad thing. Still, I'd suggest caution when using rough brushes or an exfoliating pad like a Buf-Puf. Too much friction can disrupt, you guessed it, the skin's barrier function, resulting in possible irritation, redness and increased reactivity.

Overusing abrasive scrubs can cause similar problems. Some products in this category are aggressive abraders. The exfoliating action is provided by ground-up fruit pits, nutshells or particles of aluminum oxide. I consider these rough-edged particles to be too abrasive for repeated and regular use on the skin.

But at least the fruit pits and nutshells are biodegradable. Comparatively milder exfoliant products act with round beads made out of polyethylene. Another approach is to use granules of sodium tetraborate decahydrate, a substance that softens through the exfoliating process and eventually dissolves.

The polyethylene beads are problematic because they don't break down after use. Many of them end up in oceans and lakes, where they can transport toxic pollutants up the food chain. They can also disrupt the digestive systems of zooplankton, a basic form of food for many ocean animals. The use of polyethylene beads in cosmetics has been banned in some jurisdictions.

Vitamin A Derivatives and Alpha Hydroxy Acid

Besides abrasive scrubs, another way to exfoliate the face is through what's known as chemical peels—beauty products that, through chemical and biological action, prompt the skin to shed its top layer, renewing the external skin. These products are said to reduce existing wrinkles and sun damage, fight the development of new wrinkles and in general provide the applied area with a healthy glow.

Vitamin A has two forms that occur in nature: retinol and retinyle palmitate. Other synthetic prescription forms include tretinoin (Retin-A), tazarotene (Tazorac) and adapalene (Differen). Alpha hydroxy acids—which include glycolic acid, lactic acid and salicylic acid—are used to moisturize, to exfoliate and to treat acne and psoriasis, among other uses. They work by dissolving the bonds connecting the skin cells in the stratum corneum, the outer layer of the epidermis. Low concentrations, which range between 4 and 10 percent, are used as wrinkle fighters. Higher concentrations, particularly those higher than 20 percent, are used expressly to chemically exfoliate the skin. Alpha hydroxy acids may also trigger the growth of new skin cells, which in turn is thought to boost collagen and elastic fibres and, overall, to thicken the skin layer, reducing wrinkles.

I'll discuss the many cosmetic benefits of these products in Chapter 9. But the difficulty of using both vitamin A derivatives and alpha hydroxy acids is that they can cause skin irritation. And it's a bit of a devil's bargain: The higher the acid concentration, the stronger the beneficial effect—and the more likely the product will irritate the skin. The result is red and flaky skin, as well as a burning sensation. That's okay if the reaction is temporary, lasting only 5 or 10 minutes. But in some people the irritant effect is longer lasting. If you already have reactive, irritated skin, then you should avoid these acid-based treatments until your condition improves.

I suggest that my patients begin using these sorts of products at low concentration, just one or two days a week. Once they've established that their skin can tolerate it, they can increase the concentration and frequency of use—backing off immediately once irritation occurs.

Shampoos and Conditioners

I call shampoos the hidden trigger. They're used to clean the scalp of oil as well as sweat, old skin cells, styling products and pollution. Until the mid-1930s, only bar soap was used to clean hair. Adding coconut oil to the ingredient mix created liquid shampoos, which quickly dominated the market because they lathered and rinsed better than the old bar-soap shampoos.

Shampoos are basically liquid cleansers that use synthetic detergents. The most common detergents are sulphates with names like sodium laureth sulphate, sodium lauryl sulphate, TEA lauryl sulphate and ammonium laureth sulphate. On top of these, the personal-care product industry has added many other ingredients to achieve an aesthetic result, namely boosters, thickeners, moisturizers, fragrances and antioxidants. Some shampoos even have sunscreens in them!

The problem is, the more ingredients in the product, the greater the chance that it will cause a reaction. My clinic has seen an enormous increase in shampoo-triggered reactions over the years. The majority of patients aren't allergic to things in their shampoos, although one of the ingredients that *is* causing a huge allergy problem is MI, which I discussed in the allergy section. My contact allergy colleagues and I see several patients a week who are having allergic reactions to the MI in their shampoos.

The classic shampoo-triggered reaction is a recurrent facial rash, which can be itchy, red and painful. A rash on the back of the ears, on the sides of the neck or on the shoulders is also a classic manifestation. (If you're allergic to something in your shampoo, your reaction will be severe. If your skin is just getting irritated, the reaction will be mild.)

That's why I've developed a certain relationship with shampoo. It isn't love-hate. It's hate-hate. Have you read the ingredient list on that bottle in your shower? Many shampoos contain several dozen components. Detergents, fragrances, botanicals and the dreaded MI—all of them work together and are apt, in conjunction, to cause a reaction.

Case in point: Susan, a long-term patient of mine, has rosacea, a condition of unknown cause that leads to redness, flushing and bumps on the face. We'd worked together over the years to control the condition. But lately Susan had been getting a nasty flare-up on her face.

"What changed?" I asked her. She said she'd begun using Nioxin shampoo to combat the thinning of her hair. Some detective work revealed that the menthol in the Nioxin was triggering her rosacea. Mint, peppermint and menthol are all related ingredients. They're perceived as invigorating—but can also be quite irritating. Susan quit using that type of Nioxin, and the flare-up subsided. Note that Susan's reaction wasn't allergic, but irritant.

Why would shampoo cause the eyelids, the face as a whole and the neck and shoulders to flare up—and not the scalp? Turns out that the scalp is quite resistant to immediate irritation. But the eyelids, the cheeks, the back of the ears, the neck—these parts are comparatively sensitive.

Most dermatologists consider recurrent dermatitis on the eyelids and neck to be a shampoo reaction until proven otherwise. That's why I call shampoo the hidden trigger, for irritant and allergic reactions alike. Many sensitive-skin reactions on the face, neck and upper body come from shampoo, particularly when the patient already suffers from a pre-existing skin condition, like eczema, recalcitrant itchy scalp or seborrheic dermatitis, known as dandruff.

Patients don't realize that, when they're rinsing off their shampoo, they're basically applying the stuff to every bit of skin where the shampoo sluices down. The detergents used in hair care products are also more aggressive than facial cleansers. Constant exposure can cause irritation to accumulate over time, resulting in rashes and other reactions.

Another problem is a condition known as "sensitive scalp." Compared to the eyelids and the backs of the ears, the skin of the scalp is tough to irritate. But when a skin reaction *does* occur on the scalp, it can be remarkably difficult to treat. Patients who come in complaining of a hypersensitive scalp are some of the most frustrating cases I have.

The condition, which features itchy, burning or "crawling" sensations on the scalp, is more common than you might think: In 2008, the French dermatologist Laurent Misery conducted a survey to examine the prevalence of sensitive scalp. He concluded that more than 40 percent of French men and women suffered from the condition. That's higher than what I encounter in my own practice. Still, over my 20-year career as a dermatologist, the number of sensitive scalp patients I see has increased dramatically.

Most of these patients don't have any visible rash. What's caused their condition? Overfrequent shampooing seems to be the most likely factor. From Dr. Laurent Misery: "Triggering factors of scalp sensitivity were heat, cold, pollution, emotions, dry air, wet air, water, and mainly shampoos. . . . Shampoos are triggering factors in 49 percent of scalp sensitivity."

To treat such cases, I run them through a version of the product-elimination diet that's custom-catered to the scalp. I'll describe that in the next chapter, but basically it entails switching their hair care products to fragrance-, botanical- and sulphate-free shampoos and conditioners. I also allergy-test them. Typically, they're not allergic to anything.

A small percentage of these patients continue to complain about the problem, however. I end up treating them for paresthesia—a fancy medical term that simply means "abnormal sensation." They may have permanently altered their skin's nervous response, likely through overwashing and overfrequent product use. Consequently, they need oral medications for neuralgia, which is pain or discomfort related to the nerves.

One final word about fragrance-free shampoos. Most of the brands out there tend to smell medicinal. I may not have a single person in my practice who likes to use a fragrance-free shampoo, me included. So people turn to natural, all-organic shampoos—which you know by now also can be an issue because many fragrances are natural.

I'm not telling you to join the "no-poo" movement. That's the subculture of people out there who have just plain stopped ever washing their hair. For most people, after weeks or even months, the hair apparently ends up regulating itself and looking about the same, if not better, than it did when it was shampooed regularly.

So what to do? If you have no reaction to your shampoo—great. The trick is to find the one that works for you. I admit that I myself use a fragrant, lovely-smelling shampoo, but it took me a lot of effort to find one that worked for me. And if I travel and forget to take it along, the hotel-supplied product will give me an itchy face the following day. I'll talk more about how to handle shampoos and conditioners in Chapter 6.

THE PROBLEM WITH AVEDA

Whenever I'm sent a patient with persistent itchy scalp for allergy testing, my first question tends to be, "Do you use Aveda?"

Aveda shampoos smell amazing. And they have no shortage of ingredients: Shampure, for example, has 33 listed, and that's not counting what's in the fragrance. It has such allergens as geraniol, linalool, citronella, limonene and lavender, each of which also can be irritants.

All those ingredients create a powerful scent bouquet. And thanks to recent advances in chemistry, fragrances can last for hours, as I mentioned earlier. More than any other product, the one that you can smell across the room is Aveda Be Curly Shampoo. The company says that its "pure-fume" aroma is created with "certified organic lemon, bergamot, orange and other pure flower and plant essences." All of which are potential irritants!

I often wonder if patients who use Aveda shampoo and sit in an open-concept workspace think their co-workers appreciate smelling their shampoo from across the room. Something to consider before you put on your fragrance in the morning or use a heavily fragranced shampoo.

The Product-Elimination Diet

Her case was one of the most disturbing I'd seen. Sarah, a first-year university student, had travelled three hours to visit me for her appointment. Her troubles had started six months before, when the Evolution of Smooth (EOS) brand of strawberry lip balm she was using had triggered some sort of a reaction around her lips. (I talked about this lip balm in Chapter 5.) In my office, Sarah pulled out her phone and showed me pictures that displayed a nasty rash and severe crusting.

The poor girl had stopped using the EOS balm, but the reactions had continued. They'd spread to her face and neck. We're talking severe skin redness. There was swelling and crusting around her eyes, neck and face.

Sarah had also stopped using all facial products, and had pared back her use of other beauty products. She was using only grocery-store, food-grade coconut oil as a moisturizer and a Lush shampoo bar to wash her hair. How on earth, Sarah wondered, could such natural and organic products be causing face and neck reactions?

Her doctor, having learned of my reputation as a dermatologist who can treat rashes many others can't fix, had arranged a referral. I felt terrible for Sarah when I saw her. The reactions, she said, had ruined her first year at university. She didn't want them to ruin her second year, too. Was there anything I could do for her?

First I looked up the ingredient list for the lip balm, which I expected would contain its share of allergens and irritants—since many natural beauty products do. The EOS product contained a lot of things that set off my radar. The candidate most likely to cause a reaction was linalool, a fragrance ingredient found naturally in peppermint and lavender as well as a multitude of other plants.

Next, I looked at the Lush shampoo bar, which advertised itself as specifically created to soothe irritated scalps. The marketing for this brand of bar said that it was cruelty-free because it avoided animal testing. It's great that the shampoo avoided animal testing— the world's a better place with cruelty-free beauty products. The trouble was, the shampoo bar was being very cruel to Sarah's skin. The bar contained peppermint and cinnamon. How are peppermint and cinnamon, two of the most irritating natural ingredients around, good for soothing irritated scalps?

Meanwhile, I suspected the problem was the single common denominator in the two products' ingredient lists: linalool. Recall that linalool is one of the 26 fragrance allergens the EU requires companies to include on their ingredient list. The oxidized form of linalool seems to be what's most allergenic, and the Lush soap bars definitely would have experienced enough exposure to oxygen for the linalool to become oxidized. Sarah's reactions were so bad I figured she must be allergic to linalool.

I ordered a raft of allergy tests for Sarah. But it takes a long time to get an appointment for an allergy testing session. Sometimes months. And when you do get in, you ideally attend multiple appointments within the space of a week. The tricky thing about

Sarah's case was that she had to go back to school . . . three hours away. So I scheduled her for the allergy tests the next time she'd be back in Toronto, in several months. In the meantime, I put her on the product-elimination diet—and within days, her rash improved. A patch test later that summer confirmed Sarah's allergy to linalool.

Once again, the product-elimination diet saves the day. It happens a lot. The product-elimination diet has become the centrepiece of my practice. It works for even the most problematic patients. They go home from one of my appointments and begin carrying out my advice. I hear from them soon after—because they're improving so quickly. They've been suffering for so long that they get into a near-euphoric state when they finally clear up.

They send me emails or call me up to thank me for changing their lives. And that may be so—I may have changed their lives. At least, the product-elimination diet did. But there's nothing brilliant or genius about the diet. In fact, it's a basic three-step process that anyone can do when they encounter skin problems. It's easy to do at home, and it's likely to solve most product-triggered skin problems you have.

————

Here's how I developed the product-elimination diet.

It started as something I'd get my patients to do while they waited around to be screened for allergies, which, as I said, can take months. In the meantime, I thought, why not have them avoid the chemicals that are most commonly associated with allergy and irritation in skincare? Shouldn't that help my patients' skin?

Of course it did. "I'm getting better," they'd say, and then they'd tell me they wouldn't need the allergy testing that had started the whole process in the first place. (I usually like to patch-test them anyway, since it's good to know whether they're truly allergic or just getting irritated.)

Each type of doctor has a particular clinical scenario they dread encountering. For orthopedic surgeons it's likely non-specific back pain—because the causes can be numerous and it's tough to provide the patient with a satisfying "cure." The same is true for dermatologists who encounter patients complaining of scaly skin and redness on their eyelids, which comes and goes—there some weeks, gone others.

Most of these "scaly eyelid" cases are women. At one point in my career I began encountering these patients by the dozens. Early on I would allergy-test them, and about 80 percent of the time the results would come back negative—the women weren't allergic to anything.

Take Mary, who was sent to me for allergy testing because she kept getting a red and scaly rash on her upper eyelids. Hers was a classic case. Some days the rash wasn't there. Other days, it would appear and stay for days afterward, like an unwanted houseguest. "I don't understand what's going on," an exasperated Mary told me. "I don't change my products or anything." Mary washed her hair just twice weekly. She conditioned it once a week. She did a mask once a week, and engaged in various other weekly facial regimens.

Another factor that played into what was happening: Mary was asthmatic, which meant that she had some sort of a gene or hereditary tendency for atopy, the family of immune-system disorders that includes asthma as well as eczema and hay fever. The skin of people with atopy tends to get irritated easily.

This wasn't a case of allergy. If Mary was *allergic* to one of her beauty products, the rash should happen every single time she used it. So *irritation* was the cause.

What likely was happening was an *accumulated* irritation that provoked Mary's genetic tendency toward eczema. It wasn't just one product that was bugging her skin. Rather, it was the combined effect of several products, likely working in conjunction with some other, more random factor, which could be anything from lower humidity to a particularly hot and humid day. An airborne irritant, like volatile fragrance molecules or household cleaning products, also could trigger her reaction. All of it together tipped the balance of Mary's skin irritation tolerance and created some mild redness and dryness on her eyelids—the part of the body where the skin is thinnest, and most sensitive. Bear in mind, though, that these types of scenarios can occur almost anywhere on the skin.

Think of it this way. Some days, circumstances like stress, noise and lack of sleep result in a headache. People often don't wonder *why* they get a headache—they just take a Tylenol. Similarly, the abuse to which we subject the skin—the washing and frequent product use—can provoke a rash. If that happens once in a while, just take some hydrocortisone to settle it. But if the rash, that headache for the skin, happens with increased regularity, see a dermatologist who specializes in patch allergy testing. Until then, I'd suggest the product-elimination diet.

Because here's the problem with these irritation cases. Unlike with allergy, where various types of tests allow doctors to definitively say "You're allergic to X," there's no diagnostic test for irritation.

The best way to treat any suspected case of skincare allergy or irritation is to stop using your old products and switch to my suggested list of non-irritating, low-allergenic products, set out below. Then, once your rash has cleared up, you can begin reintroducing one product from your old skincare regimen at a rate of one per week. That's basically the product-elimination diet.

This chapter outlines the process I take my patients through each time they show up with reactive skin. If you *don't* have skin issues and just want to maintain healthy skin, use this chapter as a resource. For example, if you want to use simple products that have little likelihood of causing a skin reaction, this chapter features a list of products in various categories that will provide you with some good choices. Why tempt fate with ingredients that could lead to allergy or irritation?

BOTANICALS CAN BE FRAGRANCES

Helen, who lived in a city in southwestern Ontario, came to me in desperation because it seemed as if no one could help her. Her dermatologist had discovered through patch testing that she was allergic to fragrance and plants from the Compositae family—discussed in Chapter 5, and including things like feverfew, laurel oil, yarrow, chamomile and marigold. So Helen was trying to avoid products containing those substances, except that she continued to suffer from itchy and red rashes on her eyes and ears. Sometimes her neck flared up as well.

When people with skin allergy reactions aren't getting any better, the cause is usually exposure to an allergenic substance in something they haven't yet considered.

Helen's dermatologist had given her a list of the plants in the Compositae family, with the warning that she should avoid them. She was also told to use fragrance-free skincare and beauty products. So like a good patient, Helen went out and bought fragrance-free shampoo—Avalon Organics' Gluten-Free Cucumber Shampoo— and promptly began using it. "A medley of cucumber, aloe, vitamin E and plant-derived cleansers nourish and replenish hair without fragrance or irritation," says the company's own literature, which makes a lot of the shampoo's "gluten free" certification.

The trouble was, the shampoo had several botanicals in it, including calendula and chamomile, both of which are from the Compositae family of plants—the very one to which Helen was allergic. Once she quit using the culprit shampoo, her rash cleared up.

Step One: Stop Using Your Usual Products!

What a surprise! The product-elimination diet begins by eliminating beauty products! How many? How about the vast majority of them? The next step involves adhering to a list of products you *can* use. I've gone through their ingredient lists and verified that they actually are non-irritating and hypoallergenic. For now, though, cut out your normal shampoo. Quit using your usual skin cream. No makeup. No body wash, and no exfoliant.

Stop using all the stuff you used to use!

Some women look like they want to cry when I tell them to stop using makeup. "Why do I have to stop using *every* skin, hair and nail product?" they ask me.

The answer is that some products that *seem* site-specific actually transfer to other parts of the body. And remember the study I mentioned in Chapter 3, the one that analyzed the surface of the skin and discovered that skincare products leave behind residue for days afterward?

I often get women coming back with the same eyelid, facial or body rash that caused them to visit me in the first place. "Did you stop using all your products?" I ask.

"Well," they say, if they're dealing with an eyelid rash, "I stopped all my *eye makeup*." Or they changed it to something labelled as hypoallergenic—which we both know now usually doesn't help.

The issues keep happening because your facial cleanser, *and* moisturizer, *and* hair care *and* skin and hand care can all touch your eyelid skin. Even your nail polish touches your eyelid skin. (That's actually interesting. True allergy to nail polish won't cause a problem on your nails—or even the skin around your nails. Rather, it most often creates a rash on the eyelids and neck.)

Shampoo is another product that commonly spreads itself around the body. People think shampoo would cause a reaction only on the scalp. But most shampoo-triggered reactions don't start there; as I mentioned earlier, the scalp tends to be more resistant to reactions. Shampoo ingredients rinse from the scalp on down the face and neck, and then over the rest of the body. So shampoo doesn't just affect your *hair*. That's why many shampoo products will affect the eyelids and neck before they irritate the scalp.

Or take body moisturizers. They're put on the body with your hands—and then get on your face when you touch your face with your fingertips or palms. An irritating ingredient may not provoke a reaction on your forearms or shins, but when the same fingertips that applied the stuff touch the eyelid, then a rash can result.

So, the most important first step is to stop *everything*. Regardless of where your recurrent skin reactions occur.

Just like a food-elimination diet, you have to go all in—or nothing. You have to *commit*. You can't do this on some days and not others. You can't use products on *one* part of your body and not another. If you have a facial skin issue, you have to avoid all the things on the list for *all* your body—not just your face. But don't panic, it's not forever!

So when I say restrict your use of skincare products to the things on the list, I mean it. And that includes everything: Hair products, face products, body and hand products!

One quick caveat: You may not be the only one who needs to stop using all skincare and beauty products. I've had some patients struggling with sensitive, reactive skin who have contracted skin reactions *from their partners*. A husband, say, who reacts to his wife's face cream. Face washes, body washes and moisturizers of all kinds have been known to trigger partner-to-partner reactions. So if you're romantic with someone and leaping into the product-elimination diet, you might consider asking your partner to join you—or refrain from intimacy as you go through the process.

PRODUCTS TO STOP USING

1. Hair care products, including shampoos, conditioners, mousse, gels, oils, rinses, perms, hair dyes and colouring (this is most important if you're getting rashes on your eyelids)
2. Facial products, including eye drops (unless medicated)
3. Body and hand soaps, cleansers and moisturizers
4. Makeup
5. Nail care products and polish
6. Perfumes, colognes and aftershave
7. Shaving creams or lotions
8. Prescription topical skin medication
9. Incense, essential oils and fragranced candles

Step Two: The Low-Contact Allergen and Irritant List

That said, you can use *some* products—but they have to be ones I've cleared beforehand by examining their ingredient lists to ensure that they're genuinely non-irritating and actually hypoallergenic. These are the products you can use while you wait for your reaction to clear up. Together, they're called the Low-Contact Allergy and Irritant List.

I came upon this idea at a meeting of the American Contact Dermatitis Society. A well-known American dermatologist and a past president of the ACDS, Kathryn Zug, presented a list of products that she called LowCAL—which stands for the Low-Contact Allergen List. I liked the play on words, "low cal" as in foods, but I also wanted my patients to avoid ingredients that were not just allergenic but also irritating. So I added "irritant" at the end and tweaked the list of products. It doesn't make for quite so nice an acronym—but on the other hand, it does work quite well.

The list is important because you can't just tell a patient to go and get a mild soap or a hypoallergenic skin cream . . . since, as we've already learned, labels like "mild" and "hypoallergenic" aren't reliable.

Many patients are tempted to substitute for things on the list. They go to the drugstore and a cosmetician or pharmacist might acknowledge that they don't carry this or that product. Then comes a suggestion to try another product. "This is from the same manufacturer," the pharmacist might say. Or, "Try *this*— it's for sensitive skin."

I'd tell a patient to use Dove Sensitive Skin Beauty Bar and she'd come back with Dove Go Fresh Revive Pomegranate & Lemon Verbena Body Wash. Which, like most body washes, has irritants and allergens—in particular the lemon verbena.

No no no no no no no.

The patients would return for an appointment no better than they were when they left. So I started adding this at the bottom: THE NAMES ON THIS LIST REFER TO SPECIFIC PRODUCTS THAT ARE NOT TO BE INTERCHANGED OR SUBSTITUTED.

Use the products on the list. The product names are *very specific*. You can't just use *anything* from companies known to cater to people with more reactive skin, like Dove or Aveeno, because these companies make dozens of products, and some of them have problematic ingredients.

Many companies design their products to feature very few allergens or irritants—and then, somewhere along the way, they make sacrifices and concessions. This is usually to satisfy consumer need for fragrance or naturals. So they'll include an ingredient like lavender or feverfew, both of which can be both allergen and irritant.

Again, the products featured below have ingredient lists that I've assessed. The makers of these products achieved what they set out to do. They nailed it—most of these products actually *are* hypoallergenic. The ingredient lists avoid allergens and irritants. The products avoid fragrances, sidestep allergenic and irritant botanicals and expel the preservatives associated with allergies.

USING THE LOW-CONTACT ALLERGEN AND IRRITANT LIST

1. Use exactly the products I suggest on the list! Remember that there are many different types of similar products from the same company. One name change on the product, and it has a different ingredient list.

2. If you can't find any of the products I've listed in a given category and are desperate for *something,* choose products that are soap-, fragrance- and botanical-free and have fewer than 10 ingredients. But I'd prefer that you just use what's on the list. If you can't find the products at your local pharmacy, search the Internet for online stores that carry them—and bear in mind that many of these companies sell direct to consumers.

3. If you've been diagnosed with rosacea, seborrheic dermatitis or atopic eczema, or some other skin malady, then you're likely on some sort of medication to treat it. That medication may be necessary to attain clear skin, so continue using it while still avoiding allergens and irritants in all other products. An exception is acne. Many topical acne medications are irritating, so I suggest you stop them while going through the elimination protocol. Occasionally, a product on my list may contain an ingredient that can be allergenic in rare cases. So many different allergens exist that it's impossible to avoid every single one. Some of these products may contain parabens, sulphates, polyethylene glycols or other chemicals that someone or other on the Internet may claim is toxic and should be avoided. Some fears about some of these chemicals are real, but others are overblown. In general, I tend to

be agnostic about whether a product features natural substances or synthetic chemicals. I'm much more concerned about allergens and irritants—and this list is designed to feature the minimum of each. Stick with the list, solve your skin problems and then try all the natural, paraben-free skincare products you like in a controlled manner—as described in step three below, which outlines how to reintroduce your old products.

Skin Cleansers

Patients often are told by their dermatologists to use a mild soap. What exactly does that mean? Dermatologists tend to mean a non-ionic detergent with a pH of around 5 to 6, which amounts to the skin's natural acidity.

That's a lot different from regular, garden-variety soap. Actual soap is pretty harsh for the skin, with a high, alkaline pH near 10 that disrupts the skin's acid mantle. The more natural soap you have in your bar, the more irritating it will be, and the more it disrupts the skin's natural acidity, the more it could alter the skin microbiome. Natural is definitely not better in this context.

So no matter how much goat's milk, olive oil or lavender is added to the bar, the high alkalinity in natural soap makes it damaging, irritating and drying to the skin. Remember that soap molecules have two ends. The *hydrophobic* end bonds with the grease and oil while the water-loving *hydrophilic* end bonds with the water. In traditional soap molecules the hydrophobic end is negatively charged, known as anionic. These negatively charged detergents are better at removing oil and dirt—but also better at removing the precious lipids in your skin barrier.

What's a lot better for people dealing with skin reactivity issues is synthetic *cleansers*, also known as detergents, rather than soaps. The least irritating versions have hydrophobic ends that are cationic—positively charged. Others don't have any charge at all on their hydrophobic end. Still others feature both a positive and negative charge. Those are known as zwitterions, and include popular beauty product ingredients like cocamidopropyl betaine, discussed in Chapter 5. These are certainly more gentle—but they've also been known to cause some allergies.

So what to do?

The best kind of cleansers for those dealing with skin reactivity issues are lipid-free. Such products have brand names like Cetaphil and CeraVe. They do contain detergents, but they're formulated without fats and don't strip the skin of the natural lipid layer that is so integral to maintaining the epidermal barrier function. Such cleansers do take some time to get used to. Some patients complain that they don't clean well. They don't foam or generate suds, and we've been socialized into thinking we need suds and bubbles to be clean. The lipid-free cleansers are so gentle that they may not get rid of body odour from the underarm or groin, for example. Their gentle quality is why they're here, on this list. Avoid natural soaps until your reactions have settled. For general skin health, use lipid-free cleansers and syndet bars for cleansing without irritating already reactive skin. Use the products listed below:

- Aveeno Moisturizing Bar
- CeraVe Hydrating Cleanser (no suds)
- CeraVe Hydrating Cleansing Bar
- Cetaphil Restoraderm Nourishing Body Wash
- Dove Sensitive Skin Beauty Bar (contains CAPB, which is why this product has been relegated to the bottom of the list)
- La Roche-Posay Lipikar Syndet (contains sodium laureth sulphate)
- Mother Dirt Cleanser

Hand Cleansers

Remember, don't use soap! And bear in mind, you may have to bring along one of these products if you're using the washroom at work or when you're out.

- Aveeno Moisturizing Bar
- CeraVe Hydrating Cleanser and Bar
- Cetaphil Gentle Skin Cleanser

Facial Cleansers

I'd suggest limiting your facial cleansing to once per night, particularly while you're trying to clear up reactive skin. A rinse is adequate in the morning. You don't have to wash your face with a cleanser in the morning because while you've been sleeping it hasn't been exposed to makeup or pollution.

- Avène Tolérance Extrême Cleansing Lotion
- Bioderma Sensibio H2o Micelle Solution
- CeraVe Hydrating Cleanser
- Cetaphil Gentle Skin Cleanser
- Facial Micellar no-water cleansers
- La Roche-Posay Toleriane Dermo-Cleanser
- Mother Dirt Cleanser
- Reversa Cleansing Micellar Solution
- Spectro Cleanser for Dry Skin

Facial Moisturizers

Cream, lotion, and fluid—the variety of options and consistencies allows you to select one according to your preference.

- Avène Tolérance Extrême Cream
- CeraVe PM Facial Moisturizing Lotion

- Dr. Roebuck's Pure moisturizer
- La Roche-Posay Toleriane Ultra Fluide

Hand Creams and Hand Moisturizers

Feel free to use the body moisturizers listed below on your hands as well.

- Avène Cicalfate Hand
- CeraVe Therapeutic Hand Cream
- La Roche-Posay Cicaplast Mains Barrier Repairing Cream

Body Moisturizers

Notice the natural oil-based options, which cost much less while providing many of the same benefits as more expensive alternatives.

- Aveeno Eczema Therapy Moisturizing Cream (Bear in mind that Aveeno has many different types of moisturizers, many of which include botanicals. Start with this one!)
- Avène TriXéra+ Selectiose Emollient Balm
- Bioderma Atoderm PP Ultra-Nourishing Balm
- CeraVe Moisturizing Cream and Lotion (the cream is heavier than the lotion)
- Cetaphil Moisturizing Cream and Lotion
- Curél Fragrance-Free lotion (a low-cost option, does contain eucalyptus, a rare allergen)
- La Roche-Posay Lipikar Baume AP+
- Mother Dirt Moisturizer
- Sunflower seed oil
- Virgin coconut oil

Deodorants and Antiperspirants

The majority of deodorants and antiperspirants have lots of fragrances. Here are some options that don't.

- Almay Sensitive Skin Antiperspirant (comes in roll-on or gel versions, both of which are fragrance-free)
- Vichy 24H Deodorant Sensitive Skin Aluminum-Free Stick
- Vichy Homme Roll-On Deodorant for Sensitive Skin

Shaving Creams

Typically, shaving creams and gels have abundant ingredients and lots of fragrance. Many also say they're intended for sensitive skin. Below are options that actually work.

- Aveeno Skin Relief Shave Gel
- Edge Ultra Sensitive Shave Gel (fragrance-free)

Sunscreens

Chemical sunscreens can be irritating to people whose skin is getting over a reactive episode. They can also be allergenic (see Chapter 5), although this is uncommon. I'll talk about sunscreen in more detail in Chapter 7. For now, these products are what I suggest should be used by people who are having facial reactions. They're all mineral sunscreens that don't have chemical filters or other additives, like botanicals and fragrances.

- Avène Mineral High-Protection Tinted Compact SPF 50
- Avène SPF 50+ High Protection Mineral Cream
- Bioderma Photoderm MAX Mineral Compact SPF 50+
- Clinique Mineral Sunscreen (comes in different versions for face and body, with various SPFs)

- La Roche-Posay Anthelios Mineral sunscreen (again, various versions with various SPFs)
- SkinCeuticals Physical Fusion UV Defense SPF 50

Shampoos

Shampoo is a tough category for the product-elimination diet. Most shampoos are heavily fragranced *and* contain many botanicals. They also tend to feature sulphate detergents, which can be irritating, as well as allergens like cocamidopropyl betaine and the glucosides. So it's difficult to find a perfect shampoo; all products seem to have one or two problems. While this part of the list isn't perfect, the big benefit here is that the products below are all MI- and fragrance-free. Note that I've labelled the ones that contain sulphates and those that contain CAPB. A final note: Many baby shampoos contain lots of allergens and irritants. Use the list!

- Curelle Hydra Shampoo
- DHS Clear Shampoo (SLS, CAPB)
- DHS Fragrance-Free Tar Shampoo (SLS, an option for dandruff sufferers)
- Ducray Sensinol Shampoo (contains SLES)
- Exederm Eczema Shampoo
- Free & Clear Shampoo
- Green Cricket Sky Shampoo (contains CAPB)
- Logona Kosmetik Fragrance-Free Shampoo (Germany)
- Melrose Everyday Shampoo Base (Australia, CAPB, SLES)
- Mother Dirt Shampoo

Hair Conditioners

Not every shampoo in the preceding list has a partner conditioner, nor does every conditioner in the following list have a partner shampoo. Why? Because some manufacturers don't make the partner product, for whatever reason. And in some instances I've reviewed the ingredient list and think it contains too many irritants or allergens.

- Curelle Conditioner
- DHS Conditioning Rinse with Panthenol
- Exederm Eczema Conditioner
- Free & Clear Conditioner
- Green Cricket Sky Conditioner
- Melrose Everyday Conditioner Base
- Paula's Choice Smooth Finish Conditioner

Hairsprays and Hair Gels

Besides the products below, another option you may consider while struggling with a skin reaction is not using any hairspray or hair gel at all.

- Bumble and Bumble Defrizz
- Clinique Non-Aerosol Hairspray
- Free & Clear Firm Hold Styling & Finishing Hair Spray for Sensitive Skin

Laundry Detergents

That's right—those with reactive skin should avoid the fragrances in most commercial laundry detergents. Some laundry detergents also contain the dreaded MI, so beware! Rather, opt for fragrance-, dye- and MI-free alternatives, such as:

- Cheers Free
- Ivory Snow
- Nellies All-Natural Laundry Soda Tin
- Tide Free & Gentle

Laundry Fabric Softeners

Another skin-friendly option is to dispense with fabric softener altogether and instead opt for anti-static reusable balls that tumble about in the dryer with the clothing—which have the added advantage of being friendly to the environment.

- Bounce Free & Gentle Fabric Softener Dryer Sheets
- Any dryer sheets that include the term "fragrance-free"

———

A few final notes about the products that will get you back to baseline. My female patients often ask me about what sort of makeup they should be using during the product-elimination diet. To which I reply: None! You have to avoid makeup for at least two weeks. Once their skin reactions have cleared, I steer them toward fragrance-free and oil-free products. Don't use eye shadow with mica, which is the substance that makes most of them shimmer. Matte and earth tones for eye makeup are better. That is, browns are better than purples, pinks and blues. Avoid liquid eyeliners and lip liners, which have preservatives in them. Instead, opt for pencil eyeliners and lip liners. And actually, in all things, opt for powders rather than creams or liquids. Opt for mineral-based makeups, and if you're looking for a sunscreen, go for products that avoid chemical sunscreens and instead use physical blockers like titanium. And when you're removing makeup, avoid alcohol-based removers and toners. (More on makeup in Chapter 9.)

I mentioned in Chapter 5 that if you're allergic to a particular fragrance, it's difficult to know which products to avoid. Few companies in Canada or the U.S. list the specific chemicals or substances they use to create a product's characteristic odour. Rather, they simply place "fragrance" on their ingredient list, which they're allowed to do because North American cosmetics regulations aren't as strict as they are in Europe. So for patients who are allergic to fragrance, I suggest that they employ the product-elimination diet, essentially eliminating *all* fragranced products while they get their skin back to baseline.

RECURRENT UNCONTROLLED FACIAL ROSACEA

Elena told me that her skin was very sensitive; she flushed easily, and even a light breeze could redden her skin. She'd been prescribed metronidazole cream to treat rosacea—but she seldom used the stuff because she didn't like to use medication. Instead she'd been using anti-redness creams and some natural treatments for rosacea, but with minimal improvement.

Elena was also leery of anything that sounded synthetic. She favoured natural ingredients, and was adamant that she wouldn't use parabens because her mother had died of breast cancer.

An allergy test revealed that Elena wasn't allergic to anything on the North American Contact Dermatitis Group's core allergen series.

So I put her on the product-elimination diet. After we went through my list of suggested products, Elena decided that she could live with using the following paraben-free options:

- Aveeno Moisturizing Bar (to wash her body and hands)
- Green Cricket Sky shampoo and conditioner
- Dr. Roebuck's Pure moisturizer
- La Roche-Posay Lipikar Baume AP+ moisturizer
- La Roche-Posay Toleriane Dermo-Cleanser
- Topical prescription metronidazole cream

Three weeks later, Elena came in looking a lot better. Her skin wasn't as red. She said that it wasn't as irritated as it had been, and that in general she felt better. Elena may never have skin that's completely problem-free. After all, she does have rosacea. But once she's up to 80 percent, I tell her, she can begin reintroducing her old products, one per week.

Step Three: Reintroducing Products

Many of those who begin using the products on the Low-Contact Allergen and Irritant List end up using them for life. They like how bare-bones and simple they are. Another thing that's nice about them is the price—many are drugstore brands, and very cost-effective.

Others have complaints. They say, "I want more natural." Or, "I want some anti-aging products." Or, "The lipid-free cleansers don't create enough suds to make me feel clean." Some say the cleansers are so mild that they don't remove all their makeup. (One way to address that problem is to use micellar water to double-cleanse.) The complaint I understand most is the one about the medicinal smell of some of these products. So I've created a protocol designed to allow my patients to return to at least some of the products they were using before their skin reactions happened.

That said, most patients don't *want* to return to them. For some, if the reaction was a serious rash, say, it could have been traumatic, so they don't want to risk it happening again. Others have noticed that their skin feels and looks better. Radically switching up their skincare products is an opportunity to reassess what they're doing to their skin, and most of them come out the other side not using as many products as they did before. They realize that less is more.

Hair products are the ones my patients want to return to most often. People really like fragrance in their hair care. Plus, hair can be highly idiosyncratic. Some people need to use just the right combination of products or their hair looks flat or frizzy, too oily or too dry. Something, anyway.

So here's how to get back to some of the products you were using before your skin reaction. By this point in the product-elimination diet, you've stopped using all your products and have stuck with the suggestions on the list. If you do that, your skin reaction should clear within weeks—and sometimes days.

Once the reaction is gone, you can start to introduce the products from your former beauty and skincare regimen. But don't just leap into your old routine. Rather, proceed in a step-by-step fashion. Reintroduce *one product per week*.

Usually a hair product is the first thing the patient reintroduces. So let's say you go back to your old shampoo. Give yourself a full week after the shampoo's reintroduction before you add a second product from your old routine.

This applies to anything. No matter where your rash was, again, limit yourself to reintroducing one product a week. That goes for all beauty and skincare products, cleansers, conditioners and lotions, whether it's something for the hair, face, hands or body.

By waiting a week, you're giving the product time to cause a skin reaction. It may take several days for your skin to react. If you do react during that week, then you'll know it was the newly reintroduced product that caused the reaction. After all, that's the only thing that changed in your regimen. Stop using the product—and in fact, throw it away. Toss it in the garbage. That product is causing you skin problems and you're going to have to find something else to use in its place.

If no reaction happens after a week, you're free to reintroduce a second product. The following week you can introduce a third, and so on.

Where it gets complicated is when the reactions happen after the third, fourth or fifth new product. Because at that point, it may not be just the *single* new product you happened to introduce that week. It could also be the combination of products, thanks to cumulative irritation.

So how does cumulative irritation work again? You've begun the product-elimination diet. Your skin has cleared. You've reintroduced your cleanser, shampoo and moisturizer. Next: eye shadow for a week. All good. But the *next* week, when you introduce mascara, your eyelids react. The problem may not just be the mascara. Rather, it's all of it together. Your face cleanser, moisturizer and shampoo *plus* your eye shadow and mascara have triggered a cumulative irritation that gives you some minor redness and scaling on your eyelids. So you stop the mascara, keep the cleanser, shampoo, moisturizer and eye shadow and try again.

In other words, you stop using the last product you reintroduced and wait for the reaction to clear. Once it does, keep using everything you had in your rotation before that last final product. Then introduce something else. Somewhere down the line, a few weeks later, you can test out the product that preceded the reaction.

In cases where the problem is cumulative irritation, it may be necessary to pare down the number of products you're using. For this reason, you may want to prioritize the products you reintroduce. Start the reintroduction process with the products you miss the most from your old regimen. Then move on to other products that you don't like as much.

In this step-by-step, one-product-per-week manner, even patients with reactive and sensitive skin can typically work out which combination of products is best for them. And if you can't, consider making an appointment with a dermatologist to discuss your progress. You may require patch testing to learn more about the source of the reaction.

Here's one common scenario: Patients follow the product-elimination diet and go for years with great skin. They forget about that reaction they had years back. Then they receive a gift, or go away to a spa, and rather than the basic skincare products they've been using for years, they start using a *new* product—one with a cool new botanical or wonderful fragrance. And voilà, it's back to the itchiness and burning.

Listen, I love new and interesting beauty products as much as the next person. So what I would say is, try to keep as many products in your regimen as simple as possible. Limit your beauty products to those on the list, and you can have one or two things that are more fun or that have anti-aging properties, a smell you love or an effect you like on your hair or skin. "I can't live without this *one thing*," many of my patients say. "But the rest of the boring drugstore stuff I can handle."

HEALING CREAM ALLERGY

For weeks, Ben had been plagued with a severe eruption on his lower leg that had caused him to miss work. He'd been to several doctors about it. One had prescribed him an antibiotic cream. The latest doctor had Ben going to the ER every day to receive intravenous antibiotics because she thought he had a serious skin infection known as cellulitis. By the time I saw him, the entirety of Ben's left lower leg, from the shin to around the calf, was red, swollen, scaly and weepy.

"What else are you doing to treat it?" I asked.

"Tea-tree oil," he said.

In fact, he'd been applying tea-tree oil to his leg from the beginning. The problem had started when he scraped his knee. He'd cleaned the area and then applied a tea-tree oil cream to the abrasion to assist with the healing. After more than a month that saw him taking both oral and intravenous antibiotics, he continued to apply the tea-tree oil every day, very diligently. "It's all natural," he told me.

To me it was pretty clear that the problem wasn't cellulitis—rather, the poor guy was having a reaction to the tea-tree oil.

"No more tea-tree oil," I told him. I also put him on the product-elimination diet.

Ben returned a week later completely clear. A subsequent patch test revealed that he had a strong allergy to tea-tree oil.

I've seen something similar happen with Polysporin, the brand of topical antibiotic creams and ointments. Polysporin's active ingredient is bacitracin—which causes many allergic skin reactions. The most recent patch-test data from the North American Contact Dermatitis Group suggests that 7.1 percent of those screened register as allergic to bacitracin. (Interestingly, in Europe and other countries, the incidence of bacitracin allergy is very low, probably because they don't apply Polysporin to every scrape and sore.)

I don't recommend using Polysporin. First, I'm biased against anything that has such a high prevalence of allergy. Second, antibiotics of any kind should be used only to *treat* infection—not to prevent it. The body is more than capable of healing a scrape or minor abrasion without a topical antibiotic. In fact, the overuse of topical antibiotics on healing and non-infected skin has even contributed to an increase in antibiotic resistance.

Special Skin Locations

When it comes to irritation or sensitivity, some skin areas need to be treated differently. The lips and hands are such distinctive skin environments, and under such a constant onslaught from washing, products and the elements, that they require their own special considerations.

Lips

Reactions on the lips are one of the more common referrals to my allergy clinic. Once irritated, lip reactions are difficult to treat for several reasons. They're a special type of skin, part of the mucous membrane, which tends to be more sensitive already. On top of that, we use them all day long—drinking, eating, speaking. Irritate or damage a small patch of skin *on your leg* and it heals quickly—because it's sheltered by your clothing and that skin isn't really doing anything. Meanwhile your lips are right up there on your face, exposed to sun and wind, being used to talk and eat. This near-constant barrage can prevent the lips from ever healing once irritated.

One of the strangest cases of lip irritation I've encountered happened a few years ago. It was a woman who'd been referred to me because no one could do anything about her chronic lip reaction. She suffered from a burning sensation inside her mouth as well. Also pertinent to her situation was the fact that she'd recently been diagnosed with irritable bowel syndrome. I put her on the lip-specific version of the product-elimination diet (outlined below)—but after several weeks she hadn't improved at all. Allergy testing was negative, so I biopsied her lip, and the resultant skin sample showed she was having an allergic reaction to something.

But to what?

I sat her down and we went through everything that ever came in contact with her lips, including her medication as well as the food she ate and the liquid she drank. It turned out that her naturopath had given her a special tea to drink several times a week. She sent me the tea's list of ingredients—and a single ingredient solved the problem. That single ingredient was "rhus toxicodendron." Which is derived from poison ivy.

It's hard to believe, but rhus tox is a big homeopathic remedy. Several times a week, this woman had basically been drinking poison ivy tea. She was giving herself a reaction on her lips, her mouth and the rest of her gastrointestinal tract. She didn't have irritable bowel syndrome—she was drinking poison ivy! So she stopped drinking the tea, and guess what? All her symptoms disappeared.

Happily, most of my lip reactions are a lot less bizarre. The majority can be cleared up with a version of the product-elimination diet.

Take what was happening to Terry, a well-known beauty editor turned blogger who emailed me recently out of desperation. What had started her ordeal was a dinner date several weeks before. She'd eaten hot and spicy food. This was during Toronto's harsh winter, and her lips were already a bit chapped. The next morning, she awoke and her lips were swollen and red. She switched up her lip balm several times in the aftermath, but nothing worked. (The skincare companies sent her many different products to review on her blog, so she had a lot of options.) The one she'd been using most recently was a Menthol and Eucalyptus Lip Balm manufactured by the Rosebud Perfume Co.

Meanwhile she'd stopped using any makeup products on her lips and had begun using an over-the-counter steroid cream—but her lips weren't getting better. I checked out the balm's ingredients and, like a lot of lip balms, it had menthol and camphor in it—both potential irritants.

Then I put Terry on the lip version of my product-elimination diet.

LIP PRODUCT-ELIMINATION DIET

Follow the diet for as long as it takes for the reaction to clear. The usual time is anywhere between a few days and two weeks.

1. Most lip balms contain irritants. Stop using balms that feature any of the following ingredients:
   - Beeswax (because beeswax often contains propolis, a common allergen, although some companies do remove propolis from their beeswax)
   - Fragrance
   - Menthol, mint, peppermint or camphor
   - Sunscreen of any kind
   - Any other botanical from the allergen or irritant lists in Chapter 5
2. Stop all lip makeup of any kind, including lipstick, glosses and plumpers.
3. No mint, peppermint or cinnamon in your toothpaste.
4. Use plain dental floss, without any flavour.
5. Avoid mouth rinses and washes, including Listerine and Scope, both of which contain potential irritants and allergens.
6. Stop using any chewing gums, mints or lozenges.
7. Treat the inflammation with a topical steroid cream prescribed by a dermatologist. My favourite for lips is Prevex HC, a protective dimethicone-cream base that contains hydrocortisone. If for some reason it's not possible to get exactly this product, it would help to use any mild hydrocortisone ointment prescribed by your doctor.
8. While the deeper inflammation is healing with the mild steroid cream, protect the lips' surface with a barrier cream that contains silicone, dimethicone or a variant. Use something that doesn't contain any allergen or irritant ingredients, because if you do, as I say to patients, you'll just remain in a vicious cycle of irritation. I would suggest:
   - Bioderma Atoderm Restorative Lip Balm: This is the only product I could find that contains none of the most common allergens and irritants listed in Chapter 5.

- La Roche-Posay Cicaplast Barrier Repairing Balm: Does contain beeswax.
- RoC Enydrial Repairing Lip Care: Contains several allergens and irritants, but much fewer than competing products. Allergens and irritants include methoxycinnamate, the chemical sunscreen; tocopheryl, the vitamin E allergen; and bisabolol, a derivative of chamomile.

One quick caveat, though. If you're getting only a little lip irritation every now and then, the product-elimination diet for lips is probably more than you need. Going from the typical menthol lip balm to one of the products in step 8 will likely help you heal your irritation.

The full routine tends to work for people who've tried everything else. It's for those patients who've had issues for weeks or months. They've tried many different lip balms and found that nothing worked to help their lips. They may have even visited a dermatologist and tried a steroid cream—and still they suffered from dry and irritated lips.

My youngest son read this and said, "But Mom, I love my Blistex menthol lip balm! It works great!" Remember, there are no good and bad creams, balms or moisturizers. Rather, some ingredients happen to be allergens and irritants for particular people. My boy is using the Blistex without incident. It's not causing any type of reaction at all. So, honey, I said to my boy, if you find a lip balm you like and it's not triggering a reaction, then go ahead and use it!

As for Terry, she went through the above protocol and her lips cleared up within a few days.

Finally, what happens when your toothpaste is the culprit?

Tracey was a bright dentist who was allergic to fragrance mix 1 and linalool. She'd been avoiding her allergy triggers for months and had been doing well—but now she was having a problem with her lips. I suspected the problem was the mint flavour in her toothpaste.

Dental flavour is similar to fragrance. Most of the time it's some variety of mint or peppermint—and, relative to Tracey's case, peppermint oil can contain linalool.

The problem for Tracey was that the vast majority of toothpaste includes mint as a primary flavour ingredient. What was she to do?

Non-mint toothpaste varieties aren't common—but they do exist. Flavours include strawberry, citrus, bubble gum and fennel. Here are some favourites that I suggest to patients:

- OraNurse Unflavoured Toothpaste (U.K.)
- Tom's of Maine fennel toothpaste

Once she switched to a non-mint toothpaste, Tracey's lip reaction cleared up within days.

USE HAND CREAM ON YOUR LIPS

Next to shampoos, I find lip balms to be one of the skincare market's most challenging segments—because so many lip products feature allergens and irritants. The Bioderma Atoderm Restorative Lip Balm is the best—but it can be difficult to find, as can some of my other suggestions. Keep in mind that you can source a lot of these products online.

The really important lip-protecting ingredient in barrier creams is dimethicone, a form of silicone—which is comparatively easy to find in *hand creams*. Why is dimethicone so important for lips? Because we're constantly licking, eating and drinking. If you don't have a barrier against these onslaughts, your lip irritation won't heal. Once your lips are better, use something silicone-free if this ingredient bothers you.

Try any of these hand creams to protect your lips:
- Avène Cicalfate Hand
- CeraVe Therapeutic Hand Cream

- Cetaphil Barrier Cream
- La Roche-Posay Cicaplast Mains Barrier Repairing Cream

Empty out your Blistex jar, replace it with one of the above products and feel free to use it all day long.

Hands

Hand dermatitis—a rash on the fingers, palm or back of the hand—is one of the most common referrals to my dermatology clinic. It's also the most common reason people come to the Occupational Skin Disease Specialty Clinic in St. Michael's Hospital in Toronto, where I'm a consultant for the Workplace Safety and Insurance Board.

I see hand dermatitis all day long. One recent study estimated that anywhere between 2 and 10 percent of people will develop a hand rash at some point in their lives, with the problem afflicting twice as many women as men.

We use our hands in numerous ways throughout the course of a day. In this way, the hands are similar to the lips—they're constantly exposed to the elements as well as many other things. The hands encounter soap and water more than any other part of the skin. Add the exposure to household cleaners, dish soap, shampoo and conditioner, and it becomes clear that the hands contact numerous irritants and allergens every day. And for some people, that accumulated irritation hits a certain threshold and creates a scaly, red and itchy rash—active dermatitis. "My hands have been dry for a long time," my patients will tell me. "And then all of a sudden, they got red and itchy." Or they developed deep skin cracks, known as fissures.

When I see patients with recurrent, intermittent hand dermatitis in my clinic, I like to patch-test them to rule out allergy. And while they're waiting for the patch testing—which, again, can take months—I'll put them on the hand version of the product-elimination diet.

First, I'd suggest avoiding all hand products with irritants and allergens—meaning hand soaps, moisturizing creams and the like. If that doesn't work to lessen the rash, I'd suggest moving on to the full product-elimination diet, which entails eliminating all potential irritants the hands contact, including shampoos and conditioners.

HAND PRODUCT-ELIMINATION DIET

1. Stop using all hand soaps and cleansers that are fragranced, are heavily foaming or have antibacterial ingredients.
2. Decrease exposure to water, which dries out your hands. When your hands must be dipped into water, protect them with latex-free, accelerator-free reusable gloves. I like Mr. Clean Bliss Premium Latex-Free Gloves.
3. Stop using all hand moisturizers that contain any of the allergens and irritants listed in Chapter 5.
4. If the rash on your hands is red, scaly and itchy, ask your doctor about prescribing you a topical steroid ointment to decrease the skin inflammation, which may be necessary to get you back to baseline.
5. To cleanse your hands, use the following products:
   - Aveeno Moisturizing Bar
   - CeraVe Hydrating Cleanser or Bar
   - Cetaphil Gentle Skin Cleanser
6. To moisturize and protect your hands, use a protective hand cream that contains dimethicone and does not contain allergens or irritants, such as:
   - Avène Cicalfate Hand
   - CeraVe Therapeutic Hand Cream
   - La Roche-Posay Cicaplast Mains Barrier Repairing Cream

Bear in mind that throughout the hand product-elimination diet, you'll still need to maintain the hygiene necessary to break the chain of infectious disease transmission. Rather than cleansers and water, use antibacterial hand sanitizers, which are less irritating to the skin—more on this in Chapter 7.

LATEX ALLERGY DOESN'T GIVE YOU HAND DERMATITIS

I often have patients coming in with nasty rashes on their hands, complaining that they're allergic to the latex in their rubber gloves. But here's the thing: The latex in rubber gloves comes from the rubber tree, the *Hevea brasiliensis*. Allergy to latex can cause asthma, runny nose or itchy eyes, as well as anaphylaxis—but it does not give you a scaly, itchy rash on your hands. What *can* give you that rash is a different family of chemicals, known as accelerators, which are used to speed up the rubber-making process. So to avoid such allergies, look for latex-free, accelerator-free reusable gloves for all your household or occupational needs.

Note: Beauty and skincare product ingredient lists are apt to change without warning. Also, companies introduce and discontinue products all the time. Most of the products I've suggested in this chapter have been around for a long time. In an effort to help patients and consumers, I'll maintain an updated version of the Low-Contact Allergen and Irritant List at producteliminationdiet.com.

A Common-Sense Guide to Cleansing the Skin

This book has included a lot of case studies that feature my patients. Here I'd like to share a personal story that gave me a new perspective on washing.

In 2014, I joined an expedition to the North Magnetic Pole. The expedition was led by the True Patriot Love Foundation, which was founded by my friend Shaun Francis in an effort to raise awareness of and funds for Canadian military veterans once they've returned home from duty.

The objective was to accompany 12 wounded veterans as we cross-country skied 100 kilometres through one of the world's most forbidding environments. Polar bears were a legitimate danger. The organizers figured the Arctic's alpha predators wouldn't bother us because we were a large group and had the world's best watchdog, a husky known as Diesel. But just in case, the guides kept their rifles in close reach. Nights required enduring temperatures that sank to 25 below zero. And the days entailed navigating an absolutely stunning landscape of whiteness—white snow, white sky, white ice.

All told, the expedition, led by our guide, Richard Weber, was the largest ever of its kind. I was one of the many members who'd never done anything like it. When I told friends about it before I left, they'd take a moment to get over their surprise. Once they did, they had a lot of questions for me. "Where will you go to the bathroom?" they asked. And, "How on earth will you wash yourself?"

What a reflection on our obsession with cleanliness that washing would come up so early in any discussion about the trip. But the thing is, I was a bit concerned about it myself. So here's how it went: We were on the Arctic ice for eight days. I slept in a big tent with eight men and one other woman. Each night, when I clambered into my tent, I'd wipe myself down with a paper towel and a little warm water.

It's funny. I was traversing more than a dozen kilometres a day on cross-country skis. I went without a shower for more than a week. We made it to the North Pole and back—and I didn't smell. In fact, *nothing* smelled bad. Not my feet. Not my underarms. Even the tent that housed 10 adults for more than a week—that didn't smell either. I chalked it all up to the comparatively low levels of bacteria in the Arctic's frozen wasteland.

But here's what really blew me away. After eight days on the Arctic sea ice, the expedition rendezvoused with the 1945 warplane that returned us to Resolute Bay. When I stepped into my hotel I was afraid to look in the mirror. But what I saw surprised me so much that I still think about it years later. I peered at my reflection for the first time in a week and discovered that my skin was *glowing*.

For more than a week, all I'd done was use sunscreen and rinse my skin off once a day with warmed arctic snow. My hair was greasy—but my skin was the best I'd ever seen it.

Two days later, having taken my life's longest-ever hot shower and several baths, my skin felt dry and my face had a minor red-flushed tint. (I suffer from reactive and sensitive skin myself.)

One patient of mine, Norma, experienced a similar phenomenon when she went camping in the wilderness. Norma's the kind of person whose skin gets red and blotchy at the slightest provocation. Her face can't seem to tolerate anything. I tried a number of treatments with her. But she wasn't allergic to anything, so I treated her case as I would a normal rosacea: I suggested she use a non-foaming, fragrance-free cream cleanser and a similarly gentle shampoo.

One summertime visit, Norma told me she was going canoe camping in Algonquin Park, one of Canada's national treasures. She was worried about how her skin would fare in the remote wilderness. This was after my experience in the Arctic, and so I suggested she try something. "Try doing nothing," I said. "Don't shampoo. Don't wash. Don't soap up your body in the lake. If you're going to bathe, just use lake water and a cloth. I bet you'll be surprised at what happens."

Norma was game, within reason. (If she got a cut, I cautioned her, then by all means disinfect it!) So what happened? By this point in the book, you probably know. The next time I saw her, she told me that her normally blotchy, flushed complexion had undergone a radical improvement while she was in the wilderness. By the time she arrived home, her skin looked better than it had in years.

Just like mine had.

But once she returned to civilization (with its dry, central-air-conditioned environment) and took up her usual daily showering and shampooing, the blotchy redness returned.

What's the point? A certain amount of minimal cleansing, particularly of the hands, is necessary to minimize the transmission of communicable disease. But it's hard to deny that frequent washing negatively affects the skin. I hope by this time you're looking at your daily and weekly washing routines in a different way. Of course we need to clean certain parts of the body—but excessive cleaning is not healthy for the skin.

———

One final case study for this chapter. Ray is a 50-something former athlete who works in a senior position at a global hedge fund company. I know him a little bit because our kids go to the same school. He came into the clinic one afternoon in late October. We spent the first minute or two of his appointment chatting about our sons' hockey teams, and then he came to the point of his visit. He set his leather brogue shoe on the edge of my examination table, hiked up his suit pants and pushed down his dress sock to expose the whole of his shin.

Some of the skin was red and irritated. Elsewhere it was white and flaking off. Ray grimaced when he saw it and couldn't resist giving it a good scratch. "It's so itchy," he said, frowning. "Is there *anything* you can do for it?"

There certainly was. In the autumn I see patients several times a week with what Ray had. It tends to afflict middle-aged to older men when temperatures fall and office buildings activate their heating systems. I asked Ray a few key questions. "How often do you shower?"

"Once or twice a day," Ray said. "Once in the morning, and then again after I work out."

"And are you lathering up all over?"

"Absolutely," Ray said, thinking maybe the problem had something to do with his not being clean enough. "I use soap and one of those squishy things and get the soap all over my body. Why? Should I be washing more?"

"No," I said. "That's part of the problem."

"Is it dry skin? Do you have some moisturizer you can recommend?"

"A moisturizer can help—but it's the type of soap you chose, and how much you're using, that are the most important issues," I told him. "You just need to quit washing so much—and use a non-soap cleanser when you *do* wash."

In fact, it turns out Ray was showering wrong. It's incredibly common. And it can cause problems for the skin, particularly at the advent of winter, when interior heating systems dry out homes and offices, or in hot summer weather, when the dryness comes from air conditioning.

Let's pause a moment to think about something we rarely consider: how to wash. Well into the 20th century the cleanliness ritual common to most households was the weekly bath. If you were lucky, and, more importantly, wealthy, the bath happened in your own house in a room that included supplies of hot and cold water. For the less well-off, the weekly bath happened in public bathhouses. Because, bear in mind, indoor plumbing and bathtubs and showers are a comparatively recent phenomenon. It wasn't until the 1930s that most American houses featured indoor plumbing that could supply hot water, according to Katherine Ashenburg's 2007 book, *The Dirt on Clean*. In some countries, it was much later than that.

Today, according to a 16-country survey by the market research firm Euromonitor, most people in developed nations shower *daily*. In a little more than 50 years we've increased our bathing frequency by a factor of seven.

Recall from earlier in the book that true soap strips the lipids from our skin. In the 19th and early 20th centuries, this lipid stripping happened approximately weekly. It messed up the skin for a day or two, and then our biological mechanisms returned the skin to its natural state.

These days, however, with our professional classes pursuing physical fitness in its various forms, we *never* let the skin return to its former natural state. Urban professionals are out there sweating in a CrossFit gym or on a basketball court, whether at lunchtime or after work. In the morning they take a shower. And then they take another one after their workout.

Some of them get away with it. Their skin doesn't get irritated. But for others, the incremental damage accumulates day after day, week after week, year after year. Then, with age, the epidermis begins thinning out. And a problem strikes in late autumn and early winter, when the humidity drops: The skin on the lower legs becomes itchy and irritated. It's called "winter itch," although with age it can happen during any season. It's more common in older men, who tend to soap up all over their bodies and to skip the after-shower moisturizer.

These guys are using the manly soap-based bar cleansers—Dial, Irish Spring, that sort of thing—because they think the solid bars are better at removing oil and odour. As well, they may be using shampoo and conditioner twice a day! And then, when they're rinsing it off, it all sluices down the body and seems to congregate on the lower legs. Which in turn get itchy, dry and irritated—and they end up in my office.

That's why I told Ray to cut down on the washing. "That's the cure. Don't shower so much, and switch from soap to a gentler cleansing bar. And most importantly, when you're in the shower, don't wash your entire body—in fact, just wash your bits."

When I saw Ray a few weeks later at the hockey rink, he came over and thanked me. Just as I'd told him it would, the nasty rash had disappeared. Now, he said, he works out first thing in the morning, which means he showers only once a day. When he does wash he uses a non-soap syndet bar on just his groin, underarms and feet. In fact, he told me, with this new approach he felt as if he were betraying his mom, who used to scrub him silly in the bathtub when he was a young boy.

I get patients like Ray all the time. Their skin gets irritated not because something's wrong with them, but because something's wrong with the way they're washing. So let's consider the precise method by which we're showering or otherwise cleansing our bodies. The idea might seem strange. I mean, it's *showering*, how hard can it be?

But is there any other activity we do so often and yet think about so rarely? The way we wash can profoundly affect our skin. Now, there isn't a single, perfect way to wash or clean. We're all too different for that. Nevertheless, pretty much everyone could use some pointers on the activity. Here, then, are some things to remember, followed by some suggestions for how to approach another little-considered activity, handwashing.

Showers Are Better Than Baths

Lots of my patients have this idea that all they need to do to deal with their skin problems is spend a long time lounging in a bath. Particularly if the bathwater includes some sort of salt or gel. But that's wrong. Water is known as the "universal solvent" because so many things dissolve in it. Remember those lipids that are nestled between skin cells to help the stratum corneum in its barrier function? Lounging in a bath too long gives the water an opportunity to dissolve those lipids, opening up the skin membrane to potential irritants—like bath salts or the ingredients in bubble baths. This happens all the time with toddlers. A parent will bring in an 18-month-old with an itchy rash on his skin. The parent and I discuss the mechanics of the child's bathtime. "Well," the parent will say, "I wash his hair with baby shampoo and then soap up his body, rinse him off and then we play for a while."

If I wasn't a dermatologist I might be tempted to do that, too. You want to get the work out of the way before you let the kid play. But that's exactly the wrong order. You don't want your child sitting in potentially irritating soapsuds. Instead the parent should *reverse* things—playtime happens first, in clean water, and then comes the skin- and hair-washing. Rinse off the toddler's skin and hair afterward, and then it's right out of the bath. Don't let the child sit in the bath suds. Another, even better approach to bathing a child is to use a hand-held shower wand. After playtime is over, let the water drain out; as it's draining, wash with minimal syndet cleanser and fragrance-free shampoo, then rinse with the shower wand. I discuss children and babies in more detail in the next chapter.

But Showers Aren't So Great Either

People love the shower. Particularly when it's cold out. I get it. I mean, I'm Canadian. Who doesn't love steam and hot water boosting the core temperature after you've frozen in the snow? Even the U.S. Centers for Disease Control and Prevention (CDC) acknowledges the comfort of showers. "Frequent bathing has aesthetic and stress-relieving benefits," the CDC notes, "but serves little microbiologic purpose." The little jab at the end is there because showers don't actually remove many germs from the skin.

What showers *do* remove, especially when they involve steaming hot water, is the skin's natural lipids. Which impedes the skin's barrier function, and in turn can create a vicious cycle that sees soap causing more damage, stripping out even more lipids from the epidermis and worsening the chapping caused by overfrequent and overlong showers. Which also alters our microbiome. So instead, limit the time you spend beneath that overhead nozzle. Keep it under 10 to 15 minutes, and because hot water strips more lipids than cold, reduce the temperature. Finally, try to avoid showering every day. How much is enough? There's no study on that, and everyone is different. But think about it—if all you do is go to work and sit in an office building and go home and relax, are you dirty? Do you really need a shower?

Toss That Traditional Soap in the Trash

Soap's chemistry is pretty remarkable. I've spoken earlier about how the hydrophobic end of the soap molecule bonds to dirt and the hydrophilic end allows the dirt to be rinsed away in water. But just as the law of unintended consequences dictates, that hydrophobic end also rinses away the lipids so crucial to the skin's protective functioning. Soap does its *intended* purpose really well. It gets dirt off the skin. But by stripping the skin of its natural lipids, it leaves it dry and more susceptible to infection. And with a pH of between 9 and 10, soap is alkaline, which can disturb the skin's natural acidity.

A newer invention than conventional soap is the so-called syndet or beauty bars, which combine around 10 percent real soap with what's typically a milder synthetic detergent. (These are discussed in detail in Chapter 6.) Most of the cleansing bars you buy in your pharmacy, with names like Dove, Cetaphil, Aveeno and CeraVe, are actually syndet bars. These damage the skin less.

Be Careful with Foaming Body Washes

With soap banished from the bathroom, some people might be tempted to head to the pharmacy aisle and buy a boatload of shower gels or body washes. Then they'll get in the shower, squeeze a thick coil onto the puff and lather up their whole body. But body washes can be even worse for the skin than soaps. Many body washes include a family of compounds called alkyl benzene sulphonates, cleansing molecules that work similarly to soap but for one major difference: They don't bond as well to the mineral ions found in hard water. Consequently, body wash foams up even more than soap—which makes it *even more likely* to strip the skin of its natural lipids.

In my experience, liquid body washes are frequent causes of skin irritation—they're typically fragranced and often have a host of lovely botanicals that make them smell great but can also trigger allergic or irritant skin reactions. I can recommend a couple of body washes, Cetaphil Restoraderm and Lipikar Syndet, if you like these more than the syndet bars. Both have mild suds and no added allergens.

Possibly the worst thing about body washes is implied in the name: They're meant to be used on the *body*. The *entire* body. Which by now you know isn't necessary to wash. Some would say that adding moisturizers to body washes helps counteract their tendency to irritate. But why bother to do it at all? It's a vicious cycle—irritate with overwashing, then moisturize to compensate. Instead, just wash your bits. If they called the stuff *bits* wash, maybe I'd like it better.

The worst is something I witness in the locker room at my gym: A woman will lather body wash all over and then leave it on while she shampoos and conditions her hair. That's too much time with detergent on your skin. No matter how much moisturizer is in that body wash. Look, I get it, people don't feel clean unless they have suds. They love getting out of the shower and having that tight-skin feeling people associate with being "squeaky clean." Decades of advertising have conditioned us to seek out that feeling. But you know what? That tight feeling is an indication that the skin's crucial natural fats and lipids have been stripped off the outer layer. It's actually a bad thing. Ban the bubbles!

Avoid Antibacterial Soaps and Cleansers

A number of reasons account for my strong feelings concerning antibacterial soaps and cleansers. Recall how important bacteria is to the skin's normal functioning. Maybe it grosses you out to think about a million microbes crawling around on a single square centimetre of your skin, but those creepy-crawlies help the immune system in numerous ways. We *need* them on the skin. And we need to quit wiping them out with antibacterial agents.

Triclosan was at one time the leading antibacterial compound used in soaps and other personal-care products. Both the EU and the United States have moved to ban triclosan from over-the-counter skincare products.

But it's still perfectly legal in Canada, where, at one time, the stuff was included in 1600 cosmetic and personal-care products. Triclosan and other antibacterial agents in skincare products tend to strip the skin of good microbes, too. "Consumers may think antibacterial washes are more effective at preventing the spread of germs, but we have no scientific evidence that they are any better than plain soap and water," said Janet Woodcock, an MD and the director of the FDA's Center for Drug Evaluation and Research. "In fact, some data suggest that antibacterial ingredients may do more harm than good over the long-term."

Occasionally I will prescribe antibacterial cleansers to certain patients, like the cyclists who come in complaining that they're getting pimples where their shorts chafe (because bacteria are travelling down the hair follicles). But in the majority of cases, given that antibacterial soaps can be allergenic, contribute to skin dryness and needlessly disturb the skin's microbiome, I'd say leave the antibacterials on the shelf.

Use Alternative Cleansers Instead

The holy grail of skin cleansing would be something that gets rid of the grease and dirt that accumulate on the skin through the course of a normal day while leaving behind the natural lipids of the stratum corneum. Beauty bars (Dove, Aveeno, Cetaphil, CeraVe) are the first step toward this. They're milder synthetic detergents with a small amount of soap in them. Even gentler are lipid-free cleansers, which don't have any soap at all. They use substances like propylene glycol or cetyl alcohol to cleanse the skin. With names like Cetaphil or CeraVe cleanser, they're what you should be using in the shower.

Here's the thing, though: Lipid-free cleansers tend not to foam at all. I've mentioned before that some patients just don't feel clean unless they have suds. They come back to me and complain, "Can't I just have a *little* bit of foaming in the shower?" I generally push my patients to use the stuff for several weeks in the hope that they'll get used to it.

I recently read a blog post by an advocate of organic skincare products who compared Cetaphil to toxic sludge. The post criticized Cetaphil because it didn't have any antioxidants, "omega-rich plant seed oils" or "skin-calming botanicals." I wanted to shout at my computer screen—that's precisely the point! We don't need "omega-rich plant seed oils," and those antioxidants also happen to be potential irritants! Cetaphil and its fellow lipid-free cleansers are the minimum amount of cleanser the skin requires to get off the bad stuff and preserve the good stuff. Use them instead of soap—and if using propylene glycol bothers you, stick with the syndet bars.

SOAPS ARE CLEANSERS—BUT NOT ALL CLEANSERS ARE SOAP

Soaps and detergents have been described as the most damaging of all substances routinely applied to skin. Use what follows as a guide to the most common varieties of skin-cleansing agents. And remember, the higher the percentage of soap in your product, the more irritating it will be and the more it will damage your skin's barrier and microbiome. Listing the categories from most damaging to least . . .

SOAP BARS

Made from a fat and lye. Highly alkaline, with a pH between 9 and 10. High likelihood of stripping your skin's natural barrier of oils. Typically, transparent glycerine bars, such as Pears, contain a humectant to counter soap's drying effects. Superfatted soaps contain more lipids, such as triglycerides, lanolin, paraffin, stearic acid or mineral oils, to return a protective film to the skin. And antibacterial soaps contain germ-fighting agents like triclosan, triclocarban or carbanile to inhibit the growth of bacteria, which in turn inhibits the production of odour.

COMBARS

A blend that tends to be about half traditional alkaline soap mixed with a synthetic detergent. These bars often also add antibacterial ingredients and fragrances—both of which I think are unnecessary. Examples include bars made by Dial, Coast and Irish Spring.

SYNDET BARS

Contain less than 10 percent traditional soap. The bars' slight acidity ranges between 5 to 7, which is close to the normal skin pH. Syndet bars also are known as cleansing or beauty bars. Most dermatologists recommend using this type of bar in the shower. The most frequent complaint about syndet bars is that they don't lather well, and hence don't remove enough oil from oily skin. Examples include bars made by such brands as Cetaphil, CeraVe, Olay, Dove and Aveeno.

LIQUID CLEANSERS

The more foam the cleansing product creates, the more negatively charged the detergent typically is and the higher the likelihood the product will dry out and irritate the skin. Therefore, in general, less suds means less damage to your skin. Can come in oil, lotion, cream or gel form. Oil cleansers are often less drying due to the added oil.

LIPID-FREE CLEANSERS

These cleansers contain no synthetic detergents or soaps, and don't require water to clean. Examples include such brands as Cetaphil, CeraVe and La Roche-Posay Toleriane Dermo-Cleanser.

MICELLAR WATER

Micellar water is one of the newest and best ways to cleanse the face. The active ingredients are tiny balls of cleansing oil molecules known as "micelles" that have been suspended in soft water. The idea is that the micelles attract oil and dirt, drawing such substances away from the skin without having to wet the face or lather anything. Micellar water can be used as a facial wash or makeup remover. These cleansers can remove an entire face of makeup without stripping away the skin's ability to act as a barrier. Apply the cleanser with an absorbent cotton pad.

Don't Clean Yourself if You're Not Dirty

You get in the shower, your lipid-free cleanser or syndet bar in hand. Do you get it all over your washcloth, loofah or puff and spread it all over your body? No way.

You don't need to clean yourself if you're not dirty. Have you been rubbing your shoulders in the dirt? Smearing peanut butter on your knees? Changing your car's oil with your abdomen? Of course you haven't. So why do you need to wash your shoulders, knees and abdomen if you don't have any dirt on them? If you're aiming to keep your skin in its natural, healthy state, wash only the parts that are actually dirty or emit some sort of odour. Meaning when you're in the shower, use cleansers to freshen under the arms and at the groin. That's pretty much all the cleansing you have to do in the shower.

Post-Workout Showers Should Be Quick and as Soap-Free as Possible

Ah, some patients say. But what about when I hit the locker room after a workout or tennis match? There's salty sweat all over my body—I need to wash *that* off, don't I?

No way! It's a fact of biochemistry that salt dissolves in water. That means salt *rinses*. All you have to do to get rid of that sweat is get under an overhead faucet and let it sluice off your skin. Condition yourself to avoid feeling as if you have to soap up your whole body. You don't. Also, as I talked about earlier, many of my clients end up showering a dozen times a week thanks to the post-workout shower. That's not good for your skin, either. To limit the number of showers you require in a week, consider skipping the one you take in the morning if you're going to get in a lunchtime workout and plan to shower after that.

Most of Us Don't Have to Exfoliate

Our skin is exfoliating itself all the time, naturally. You don't have to help the process along. As we age the exfoliation process can slow down a little bit. So if you're older, you may want to pursue some sort of physical exfoliation. That entails taking a loofah, a natural sea sponge, and rubbing it over the arms and legs in the shower. This can also be done as a dry rub, or what's called dry brushing. Don't use exfoliating scrubs—you don't need them, and they may actually exfoliate too much, irritating the skin.

Use "Simple" Shampoos and Conditioners

As I said earlier, most dermatologists consider shampoo the prime suspect for any rash on the front or sides of the neck. The issue with most shampoos is the sheer volume of ingredients they have. The more ingredients in anything, the more likely *something* is going to be allergenic and irritating to the skin. All that stuff is going all over your body. Down the drain, too. And the organic shampoos tend to contain a lot of botanical ingredients—things like mint and citrus, which can be just as irritating to skin as chemical fragrances.

The sheer volume of ingredients is the reason I find hair washing to be a much more challenging topic than washing our bodies. Technically speaking, the hair is a dead protein. It doesn't *need* to be cleansed. I like the way dermatologist Zoe Draelos puts it: "Hair does not really need to be washed. It is nonliving and does not produce sebum or sweat. It is the scalp that produces these materials that are then wicked from the scalp down the hair. Certainly, if the hair gets full of environmental dirt or food, it needs to be washed, but this is rare in adults."

That said, I *like* washing my hair. I like how my hair feels afterward. I like how it smells. Lately I've been using a dry shampoo to absorb scalp oil every three days or so. But it's tricky. If you want to play it safe, or have had issues with reactions, stick with the list of shampoos in Chapter 6. And if you don't have issues with reactive skin or scalp, feel free to experiment.

Take a less-is-more approach with product ingredients. If possible, avoid the ingredients I mentioned in Chapter 6. Be careful with allergens like CAPB and the dreaded MI. Many patients I allergy-test due to itchy scalp or recalcitrant dandruff turn out to be negative. Once I stop their shampoo with its several dozen ingredients and get them using the ones listed in Chapter 6, their skin conditions settle. Before too long they can often return to their old shampoo once the condition has stopped. Still, it's useful for these patients to go back to the non-irritating shampoos once in a while to interrupt the cycle of irritation.

COMMON-SENSE HAIR CARE TIPS

1. If your hair isn't dirty or greasy, don't shampoo it every day.
2. If your hair is long, wash your scalp, not your hair. The oil is near the scalp, and the surfactants will damage the ends.
3. Avoid sulphates, fragrances and botanicals if you have a dry, irritated scalp.
4. If you suspect an allergic reaction to MI or one of the synthetic detergents like CAPB, use the suggestions on the product-elimination diet list, page 157. Remember, these reactions often present as significant or persistent eruptions on eyelids, necks and ears, and not the scalp.
5. Use dry shampoo several times a week to decrease the amount of shampooing.

6. Use co-washes or non-detergent hair cleansers more frequently than shampoos. Be careful, though, as many contain fragrances and botanicals, which could irritate.

7. I don't think it's necessary to add oils to most types of hair. (Except for African-American hair, which can become dry due to the shape of the hair shaft.) Oil counteracts the dryness that shampoos and other hair products produce, yet it can also lead to acne on the face and neck. It's the same cycle I talked about with the skin: overwash, irritate and then try to counteract the damage with product.

Consider a No-Detergent Shampoo, or Co-Wash

One of the big trends in hair care is trading a traditional shampoo for a cleanser that doesn't contain any detergent. Known as no-detergent shampoos, or co-washes, these products cleanse your hair gently without drying it out. African-American women have been using co-washes for years because detergents are so likely to damage their hair. Now, thanks to a reluctance on the part of consumers to use products with sulphates, and an awareness that shampooing can actually damage the hair and the skin, co-washing is spreading to other sectors of the market.

Co-washes usually use some combination of organic ingredients that result in a form of cleansing. One concern I have about these new products is that many of them still have a lot of ingredients, and lots of ingredients means an incrementally greater likelihood of triggering allergen or irritant skin reactions. One product generating lots of media attention is New Wash hair cleanser from the Bumble and Bumble founder Michael Gordon, who hopes that his customers will never again use traditional shampoo. More controversial is WEN from Chaz Dean Cleansing

Conditioners, the co-wash product that's been the source of thousands of complaints to the FDA in recent years over such reactions as hair loss, balding, itching and rash. Consumer beware.

Cleanse Your Face with a Non-Foaming Facial Wash

To cleanse the face, I suggest that you stick with the products I recommend in Chapter 6. If you don't like the lipid-free cleansers, try their foaming facial variants.

- CeraVe Foaming Facial Cleanser
- Cetaphil Foaming Facial Wash
- La Roche-Posay Toleriane Purifying Foaming Cream

When trying out cleansers, take a less-is-more approach: no fragrance, dyes or allergenic botanicals. Whether you choose a cream, lotion or gel, as long as it's water soluble, the product will be either light or high foaming—and remember, the more it foams, the more drying it tends to be. Creams and oil cleansers tend to be less drying than gels. Consider the latest cleanser, micellar water, which is a great way to clean without water. Apply it with a makeup pad. Some patients like to use micellar water after their lipid-free cleansers.

When you do go from a lipid-free to a water-soluble cleanser, try to keep all your other skincare routines the same. That way, if you do react, you'll know for certain that the cause is the switch in cleansers—and it'll be easy to treat the reaction by returning to your lipid-free cleanser.

Handwashing Can Cause Problems

For all my ranting against washing, I do believe that hand cleansing is required to break the chain of transmission for communicable disease. Particularly in an age of frequent global travel. But that causes its own set of problems.

Hands feature several different environments. The palms are thick, for example, while the tops of the hands have thinner skin. Once the skin on the fingertips or palms is compromised by overfrequent handwashing, it takes a long time for it to heal. Why? Because the skin on our hands never gets a break. We use our hands all day long—to clean ourselves, prepare food, open doors, move paper. All this exposure to constant irritation prevents the skin from healing.

Hand cleansing can be achieved in numerous different ways. I'd never suggest using antibacterial hand soaps. Rather, America's Centers for Disease Control and Prevention (CDC) guidelines suggest a five-step protocol that sees you using soap and water to scrub your hands for at least 20 seconds, or long enough for two complete hums of "Happy Birthday." Here are some of the times the CDC suggests it's a good idea to wash the hands:

- Before, during and after preparing food
- Before eating food
- Before and after caring for someone who is sick
- Before and after treating a cut or wound
- After using the toilet
- After changing diapers
- After blowing your nose, coughing or sneezing
- After touching an animal
- After handling pet food or pet treats
- After touching garbage

However, following these suggestions to the letter could require that people in some professions wash their hands dozens of times a day. Which is why one of the most common visitors to my clinic are patients with incredibly dry hands. That kind of washing frequency can lead to skin dryness and cracking, which can in turn lead to infection, ironically bringing about a scenario that sees handwashing actually *increasing* germ transmission.

"The goal," according to the CDC, "should be to identify skin hygiene practices that provide adequate protection from transmission of infecting agents while minimizing the risk for changing the ecology and health of the skin."

I tell my patients to use a cleanser and water if their hands are visibly dirty. That is, covered with mud, grease, paint, ink or any of the other substances that can get on the fingers and palms through the course of the day.

But if your hands aren't visibly dirty—if you're simply concerned with germs and disease transmission—then using an alcohol-based hand sanitizer is better. Such sanitizers have the added advantage of being less likely to dry out and irritate the skin. According to no less an authority than the World Health Organization, "Of the published studies available, many describe that nurses who routinely use alcohol rubs have less skin irritation and dryness than those using soap and water." That's my experience, too. In fact, in pretty much every case I'd prefer that my patients use sanitizer rather than washing with soap and water, or even a cleanser and water. Unless you've been out in a park making mud pies, use sanitizer. Also, avoid the sanitizers that have extras like aloe or lavender—they're potential irritants and you don't need them.

Gloves are another option. I've seen food-service workers preparing a sandwich, accepting money in payment, then turning to a sink for a quick handwash before the next customer, at which point the worker repeats the routine again. In a single shift the poor worker probably washes his or her hands 60 or 70 times. Wearing a pair of vinyl gloves for the food-service side of the routine would be a lot better. The same is true for such daily chores as dishwashing or cleaning the car. Bear in mind, though, that wearing a rubber or vinyl glove of any kind for longer than 20 minutes is bad for the hands, since the sweat can dry out the skin. If you need to be in gloves longer than 20 minutes, use a thin cotton glove under the outer glove.

PROTECT YOUR HANDS WITH BARRIER CREAMS

To ward off dry hands in situations that require frequent handwashing, use a hand barrier cream rather than just a moisturizer. What's the difference? Such products as glycerine, Vaseline and shea butter do help moisturize the hands, but the effects of these products disappear quickly in those who continually assault the skin with washing through the course of a day. In contrast, barrier creams that contain dimethicone, or some other form of silicone, will wick water away from the hands, allowing your skin to heal underneath the barrier. In particular, I like:

- Avène Cicalfate Hand
- CeraVe Therapeutic Hand Cream
- La Roche-Posay Cicaplast Mains Barrier Repairing Cream

Skincare for Babies, Children and Teens

When I was a young working mother of two children, aged three and two, we happened to live beside Red Kelly, the famed hockey player and later NHL coach. One day I got to talking with Kelly. If I wanted to sell the kids on Canada's national sport, he said, then I should have the boys walk about inside while wearing black figure skates so that they could get used to the feel. (Figure skates apparently support the ankles better than hockey skates.) Game for anything Kelly might suggest, I dutifully equipped the boys' skates with blade guards and let them clump around our house for months. And it worked. Nearly two decades later, I'm a proud hockey mom. I'd go on to have another boy, bringing my total to three, and they've all excelled at the sport.

Competitive hockey kids are crazy athletes. They usually like to do multiple sports. But the thing about hockey is, it can be dangerous. The puck is rubber, hard and heavy. The ice might as well be concrete and the bodies move with speed—often into one another. Injuries are inevitable. So are dirt and the dreaded hockey odour. Few things in existence smell worse than hockey equipment.

Most would expect a mom who was an MD and dermatologist to be obsessed with hygiene—running around with wipes, always ready with the alcohol-based hand sanitizer. But if you've read this far, you'll know that wasn't me. In fact, I was the opposite of the helicopter parent. "If you're not dirty, you're not having fun" went my motto. "A little scrape or blood is okay—it means you're alive."

Sometimes when my boys were beating each other up, as boys are apt to do, one of them would come to me to complain. "Is anyone bleeding?" I'd ask. "If not, work it out yourselves."

Today we have whole books written about how we're ruining our children by being too attentive and too danger-averse—keeping them insulated from the slightest scrape and in general never exposing them to the outside world. I tend to agree with the criticism, particularly when it comes to how we take care of kids' skin.

And I am not alone. It is the dermatology community's opinion that most of us wash our children way too much. Unless your child is covered in mud or some other undesirable substance, you don't need to soap the entire body. The daily bath is probably doing more harm than good, particularly if it includes an all-over soaping. For example, the application of harsh soap to babies' skin during the first year of life may have increased the incidence of atopic eczema. "The prevalence of atopic dermatitis among babies and children has risen from around 5% in the 1940s to up to 25% today," says Michael Cork, a professor of dermatology at the U.K.'s University of Sheffield medical school. "Clearly over this period genetics haven't changed, but our environment has, particularly the way we treat babies' skin."

We're doing too much to our children, in other words. Bathing too much. Scrubbing too much. Soaping too much.

I bathed my children just three or four times a week when they were young. I'd let them play in the water first, and would use only a synthetic detergent before they exited the bath. No sitting in detergents. No bubble baths or real soap bars, or any fun-smelling shampoos. My children have a family history that predisposes them to atopic conditions, and yet my boys never developed any—that is, none of them ever had asthma, hay fever or eczema.

Did my laissez-faire philosophy on cleanliness help them avoid the atopy to which they were predisposed?

I like to think so.

In contrast, one of my good friends had lots of allergies as a child, including hay fever. Two of his three children are plagued with it; the other had atopic eczema. When those kids were little my friend and his wife were germaphobes. They washed their kids constantly—scrubbing them all over with soap, deploying an alcohol-based hand sanitizer on a moment's notice. Helicopter cleaners—that's what they were. And it may have tilted their children toward the atopy they subsequently contracted.

These are anecdotal accounts, of course, but my speculation is based on hard science. Research indicates that frequent all-over washing and the use of harsh soap and detergents play some sort of a role in predisposing kids to eczema, asthma, hay fever and other atopy-related allergies. In fact, much of the advice I'll give you in this chapter is based on advice from the American Academy of Dermatology, to which I belong.

Newborns and Babies

You've likely heard the expression "smooth as a baby's bum." There's a reason why babies' skin is so smooth: It's new. But that skin is also much thinner than what covers fully grown human beings. By its very nature, the barrier function of baby skin is compromised. It can't protect the child from the external world the way our skin does later in life.

In adults, the stratum corneum, the skin's outermost layer, has between 10 and 20 layers. In prematurely born infants under 30 weeks gestation, though, it has just two or three layers. And by the end of the baby's first year, that outer layer is still about 30 percent thinner than the adult stratum corneum. Newborn skin also has a different pH: It's comparatively alkaline, with a pH of about 6, falling to less than 5 as the baby matures. Interrupting the acidification of a newborn's skin can result in problems. Skin is designed to be somewhat acid as a way to maintain its barrier function and protect it from disease-causing bacteria. If the skin is *too* alkaline, that protective feature doesn't exist and the barrier can fail.

Another consideration is the "seeding" of the baby's skin microbiome. In utero, the fetal skin is sterile. That is, there are no bacteria on it. Just a year after birth, however, billions of bacteria have colonized the skin. Seeding is the process by which the skin goes from empty to teeming with microscopic organisms. Think of it as the colonization of an alien planet, something I talked about back in Chapter 3. It begins happening right from the moment of birth. If the birth happens vaginally, the skin is colonized by the mother's vaginal bacteria. But if it happens via Caesarean, the skin is colonized by the mother's skin bacteria, among other things—and the baby's microbiome ends up being less diverse. Scientists don't know exactly how that affects the development of the baby, but at this point we do know that less diverse microbial flora in a baby's gut and on the skin is thought to be a factor in the development of various maladies, including atopic diseases like asthma, eczema and hay fever. "Proper and early establishment of a healthy skin microbiome may affect the development of skin immune function and the development of the systemic immune system," says Joanne Kuller, a California neonatal nurse and an expert on neonatal skin.

In fact, the early development of a healthy skin microbiome is considered so important to healthy immune function and the avoidance of atopic diseases that scientists are working out some pretty unconventional ways to colonize neonatal skin. For example, NYU School of Medicine associate professor Maria Dominguez-Bello established that, in babies delivered via Caesarean, the swabbing of the baby's skin with healthy bacteria from the mother's vagina increased the diversity of the bacteria on the infant's skin.

Consequently, we have to be more careful with the skin of infants than we otherwise might. Take a ritual that happens in every baby's life: the first bath. My eldest son was born in 1999 via an emergency C-section. I was exhausted by the ordeal, and soon afterward, one of the nurses went to take my baby from me. To give him a bath, she explained. But I wouldn't let him go. There were a few things going on here. First, I just wanted to hold my baby. Second, I wanted to be the one to give my boy his first bath. And third, I didn't trust the sort of products the hospital would have.

Nearly two decades ago, the hospital may have used any number of detergent products on my newborn. This was before the research establishing the importance of the skin microbiome—and before the research establishing that soap use and overfrequent washing in that first year may play a role in the baby developing atopic diseases, such as asthma, eczema and hay fever. I used plain water and a soft cotton cloth the first few times I bathed my baby.

Nearly 20 years of research suggests that I performed my son's first bath relatively well. Here's where the guidelines stand today. Drawing on the work of Kuller and Cork, I'd suggest waiting two to four hours after birth to give the first bath. I wouldn't allow the infant to linger in the bath water. Remember, water itself is drying. Limit bathtime to between 5 and 10 minutes. Water temperature should be warm to the touch, but not hot. A little bit of mild cleanser might be necessary to wash blood and amniotic fluid from the infant's skin. Same with the diaper area.

Most of us, when we're washing, think we have to get everything off the skin. But your job with the first bath is not to give your baby a vigorous buff and polish. The emphasis here should be on making the experience soothing—bearing in mind that "soothing" may be impossible when you're an anxious, exhausted mother working to clean an infant who may be squirming in the middle of his or her first temper tantrum!

You'll want to use something for friction as you bathe the child. For that I'd suggest a soft cotton cloth or a mild wipe. But as much as possible, allow the vernix—the white, waxy stuff that covers the baby's skin—to remain on the baby, because it may help the skin's pH fall to the appropriate level.

Once you're through the first time, bathing requires some special measures for as long as the infant is in diapers. One big issue here is that during the first 12 months of life the baby's skin isn't yet mature. It doesn't protect from irritants or allergens the way adult skin does, so you have to be more careful with a baby's skin than your own. Overfrequent washing and the use of harsh cleansers on baby skin have likely played a role in that increase of atopic diseases I mentioned earlier. According to a 2014 paper, about 60 percent of babies get atopic eczema in the first year, with 85 percent of cases developing during the first five years of life. Dr. John McFadden, a dermatologist at London's St. Thomas' Hospital (whom I first cited in this book's Introduction), believes that the chemicals in toiletries, not just the detergents, can push babies' immune systems toward atopic eczema. "Chemicals" here refer to allergens and irritants rather than expressly synthetic substances. Dr. McFadden means any chemical exposed to the baby's immune system, regardless of whether it's natural or synthetic. So that would include many botanical and organic things. I agree with Dr. McFadden. Less is more when it comes to a baby's skin—it's not about what's natural.

Lots of studies have revealed the mechanism that may be at play in the development of atopy in young children. It seems to have something to do with a protein called filaggrin: Those who have a parent or grandparent with asthma, eczema and hay fever likely possess a gene that prevents the body from making appropriate amounts. In those with healthy skin, the breakdown of filaggrin creates a substance that moisturizes the skin and keeps the skin surface comparatively acidic. Without enough filaggrin, the stratum corneum cells contract and the skin surface grows alkaline, triggering a process that allows allergens and irritants to penetrate the skin's protective layer. That can lead to atopic eczema, which in turn may lead to other atopic conditions, such as asthma, hay fever and food allergies, in what's known as the atopic march.

This process seems most likely to happen before the skin matures—and protecting the infant's skin through the first years with appropriate washing and moisturizing seems to decrease the risk of developing atopy. So what's "appropriate" washing and moisturizing?

By now, it's probably unnecessary to say that I don't want you to use soap or bubble bath. Also avoid bath oils or bath "bombs." Instead, wash your baby with a mild, fragrance-free cleanser. "Wait a second," you may be thinking. "You've said throughout that we use too many soaps and cleansers—and now you're telling me to use cleanser on my baby's sensitive skin? What's up?"

It's a good point. But the thing is, plain water just can't cleanse the baby appropriately, and several studies have shown this. For one, there's the fact that tap water can have a pH of 7, or even higher if it's hard—in Toronto, where I live, the pH of tap water is 7.7. Using just plain water and a cloth to bathe a baby risks prolonging the bath, resulting in an elevation of the baby's skin pH that could compromise the barrier function.

Something else is at play, here, too. At exactly the point in the life-span when the skin is most sensitive, the baby's outer layer is coming into contact with all sorts of stuff—feces, urine, foods—that adult skin never has to deal with. So the appropriate cleanser is crucial.

But which one? The work of Dr. Michael Cork, a U.K. expert in the relationship between neonatal skin and atopic eczema, helps to narrow down the options. Cork conducted an experiment in which infants were bathed with either Ivory Soap or Johnson & Johnson's Top-to-Toe baby wash (which is sold in the U.K.). With just a two-minute wash, the Ivory Soap raised the pH of the babies' skin to 6.8, where it stayed for four hours. Top-to-Toe, in contrast, maintained the skin at a pH down around 5.7—which is a lot healthier. Cork went on to study a natural soap, Earth Mama Angel Baby, and showed that it not only increased babies' skin pH but altered the barrier function as well.

Because of such studies, I suggest using only mild cleansers and wipes during bathtime through a child's first couple of years—both to maintain an acidic pH of the skin and to assist in the removal of all the stuff you want to get off your baby. Just because the product says "baby" on it doesn't mean it's mild or appropriate for babies. Remember, labelling cannot be trusted. My favourite study to prove that was conducted in California and published in 2015. "Anecdotally," the authors write, "we have observed a lack of correlation between marketing terms highlighting hypoallergenicity or dermatologist/pediatrician-recommended status and the actual content of contact allergens in topical products." To prove their case, the researchers went out and bought 187 products that were marketed as "hypoallergenic," "for sensitive skin," "fragrance-free" or "paraben-free." They also examined products that said they were recommended by dermatologists or pediatricians. And fully 167 of the 187 products contained at least one allergen, with the average number of allergens in each product coming in at 2.4.

In addition, I'd suggest avoiding anything that contains sodium lauryl sulphate or sodium laureth sulphate, or even syndet bars like Dove, Cetaphil and CeraVe, because they can contain up to 10 percent real soap. Use absolutely no soap on babies during their first year. If I were a new mother today, here's what I'd use on my children:

- Cetaphil Restoraderm Nourishing Body Wash—Note that I'm not recommending Cetaphil's *baby* wash, which has among its ingredients sodium laureth sulphate.
- CeraVe Baby Wash and Shampoo—No fragrance or unnecessary botanicals. This product does have the synthetic detergent decyl glucoside, which can be allergenic in rare cases.
- Avène TriXéra+ Selectiose Emollient Cleansing Gel—A good cleanser with a long and complicated name. Only caveat: It does have a mild anionic surfactant, disodium laureth sulphosuccinate, but no fragrance; ingredients phenoxyethanol and vitamin E can be allergenic in rare cases.
- Aveeno Baby Soothing Relief Creamy Wash—Contains cocamidopropyl betaine, which is allergenic in rare cases, but no fragrance. This is a cream wash that doesn't create much lather—remember, you don't need suds to clean!
- Johnson's Head-to-Toe Baby Wash—A good cleanser, albeit one that includes fragrance. Also contains cocamidopropyl betaine, phenoxyethanol and ethylhexylglycerin, each of which can be allergenic in rare cases.
- Skinfix Baby Wash—For those who seek a more natural and organic option, the Skinfix product contains no sulphate detergents. It does contain decyl glucoside and vitamin E, which can be allergenic in rare cases, as well as the allergenic botanical ingredients calendula, rosemary and chamomile.
- Finally, shampoos. It's fine to use the washes listed here as shampoos. Another possible course of action is to use one of the

shampoos listed in Chapter 6. You should start this practice after
year one, though, since some of the shampoo suggestions do
contain sulphates. And avoid getting the suds on the rest of the
infant's body.

Other things to remember:

- There's a tendency to overwash babies. The new parent wants
  to be seen as a good parent, and so anytime the infant gets
  anything on his or her skin, it's into the bath. Don't feel bad if
  you don't bathe your child every day. At the same time, I'd set a
  maximum bathing frequency of three times a week.
- The most important thing to remember during those first years
  of life is to avoid soaps or cleansers that increase the skin pH—
  that is, products that contain sulphates and real soap.
- That said, use more than just water to keep the diaper area
  clean. I'd suggest a cloth and water, along with some sort of a
  mild cleanser.
- Another option is to use baby wipes to keep the diaper area clean.
  Some studies show that mild wipes are better than water, cloth
  and cleanser because the wipe alters the skin's pH less than the
  cleanser does. If you do opt to use wipes, avoid those that have
  alcohol, MI, botanicals or fragrances in them. If I had a baby
  today, I would go the wipe route and use Huggies Natural Care
  Wipes or Huggies Simply Clean Wipes from Kimberly Clark.
  Neither uses fragrances or MI but they do have vitamin E and
  coco-glucoside, which in rare cases can cause allergic reactions.
- In any products you're using for your baby, make it a goal to
  avoid unnecessary allergens. So that's things like fragrances
  and botanicals—avoid lavender and other unnecessary plant-
  based chemicals.

DIAPER DERMATITIS

Also known as diaper rash, the redness and, in worse cases, sores happen when urine and feces touch the skin for extended periods of time. A chemical reaction results: Enzymes from bacteria in the feces react with the urine to release ammonia, which then raises the pH of the skin and disrupts the skin's barrier function. To prevent diaper rash:

- Change diaper frequently during first month.
- Superabsorbent diapers are better.
- Allowing the infant to go around without a diaper—diaper "holiday"—can give the skin a break and prevent irritation.
- After each changing, apply plain Vaseline or a zinc-oxide ointment as a diaper cream.
- If irritation continues, after each changing apply a thick paste like Ihle's Paste, a 25 percent zinc-oxide ointment. Apply a layer so thick that you can't see the skin. Don't rub this in—it's meant to stay on as a barrier between the skin and the diaper contents.
- Avoid talcum powder, topical antibiotics and steroid creams.

Prophylactic Moisturization

One of the more exciting areas of pediatric dermatology is in measures to *prevent* atopic eczema in kids at high risk of developing the condition—namely, those whose parents or grandparents already have it. Atopic eczema is increasingly seen as an important stepping stone in the atopic march, which, as I noted earlier, can lead to asthma, hay fever and food allergies. Stop atopic eczema in babies and children, the thinking goes, and maybe that'll stop the related maladies that occur later in life. At this point, one of the most promising therapies involves what's known as prophylactic moisturization. It amounts to applying a dye-free, fragrance-free moisturizer all over your baby's body, except for the scalp, every day for the first six to eight months of the infant's life.

At a time when the infant's skin isn't yet mature, the moisturizer is thought to bolster the skin's barrier function—sealing the infant from the allergens and irritants that may play a factor in eczema's development.

But which moisturizer is best? I've seen studies that demonstrate the effectiveness of everything from plain old Vaseline to sunflower oil. If your baby has a family history of atopic eczema, follow the bathing rules above. In addition to that, consider applying moisturizer to your baby's skin daily through the first six to eight months of life. Most of the following products appear in my list of suggested moisturizers for adults in Chapter 6. This list of recommended moisturizers for babies and children also features natural plant oils that are neither allergens nor irritants—as well as what's likely the most cost-effective option, Vaseline. Remember: Your baby does not need lovely-smelling skincare products to get him or her to sleep.

- Aveeno Baby Eczema Therapy Moisturizing Cream
- Avène TriXéra+ Selectiose Emollient Balm
- Bioderma Atoderm PP Ultra-Nourishing Balm
- CeraVe Moisturizing Cream and Lotion
- Cetaphil Moisturizing Cream and Lotion
- La Roche-Posay Lipikar Baume AP+
- Sunflower seed oil
- Vaseline Petroleum Jelly
- Virgin coconut oil

Finally, one thing to bear in mind: Some natural oils, such as olive oil, are not good for the skin barrier. The ones listed above have had extensive studies to prove their benefit. Also, I wouldn't use coconut oil on the face, where its pore-clogging properties can cause acne, even in babies.

I would suggest not using sunscreen for babies, particularly during the first six months. Rather, keep your infant out of the sun. Cover him or her up with sun-protective clothing. Your babies and young toddlers won't care what they wear. This comes later. So dress them in full sun-protective suits that have a UPF rating, which is like an SPF rating but for fabric. Also use sunhats with flaps! After the first six months until two years old, avoid sun exposure between the hours of 11 a.m. and 3 p.m. When on holiday, or if you live in a warm climate and your kids are swimming or out all day, get a full-body sun-protective swimsuit or long-sleeved UPF shirt and a hat with a wide brim (not a baseball cap). At other times, I'd suggest a mineral sunscreen with an SPF of 50+. I prefer to avoid the chemical sunscreen ingredients until the age of two. My favourite is Avène Mineral Cream SPF 50, as it stays on very well and gives excellent protection. I used it on all my children.

Children (Aged Two to Puberty)

Most kids bathe too much. My generation grew up at the height of the daily bath ritual. Our mothers insisted not only that we take a bath every day but also that we wash ourselves everywhere, with soap, including behind the ears. They inspected the backs of our necks for grime. And the practice was terrible for our skin.

We've known this for a long time—but it's just beginning to percolate up from the academic literature through to the medical profession and on to the populace at large. One of the key studies that established it also happens to be one of my favourite academic studies ever. It's called the Avon Longitudinal Study of Parents and Children, also known as the Children of the 90s Study. Researchers from the University of Bristol tried to gather as many pregnant women as they possibly could in the years 1991 and 1992. All told, they mustered 15,247 pregnant women—and then studied the children after birth in an attempt to determine how their lifestyles affected their health in the ensuing years. The study has answered all sorts of questions about how best to care for babies and children. And one aspect of this study, the one that's most pertinent to this book, involves the optimum frequency of bathing.

When the children were 15 months old, the researchers asked the parents about the way they washed them. Among this group of children in southwestern England, most, approximately 55 percent, were bathed every day. About 5 percent were bathed at least twice a day, 36 percent several times a week, and just 4 percent once a week or less.

Then the researchers followed the children. For years. And they discovered that, in general, the cleaner the kids were—that is, the more obsessed the parents were about keeping them clean—the more likely they were to develop eczema and asthma. To state the findings another way: The more baths the kids had per week, the higher their risk of developing eczema and asthma. And further research has borne out this conclusion, suggesting a causal relationship between overfrequent bathing and risk of developing atopic diseases.

Not only that. There are good indications that the incidence of pediatric allergic contact dermatitis—rashes caused by exposure to things that come into contact with children's skin—is increasing. Guess what I think is the best explanation. That's right: overwashing and overfrequent product use at a younger age. The application of too much soap on children's skin, too frequently. And when skin reactions or atopic eczema do occur, parents rush out to buy products marketed as "hypoallergenic" or targeted for those with "sensitive skin." And by now we all know how unreliable such marketing can be. Many such products are loaded with fragrances, botanicals or surfactants, from cocamidopropyl betaine to beeswax, that can cause allergenic or irritant reactions.

In fact, the harmful effects of overwashing children have become so firmly accepted that in 2016 the American Academy of Dermatology released bathing-for-children guidelines that would have sounded, to parents of previous generations, like neglect. Bear in mind, this isn't an outlier organization. The American Academy of Dermatology represents 18,000 skin-focused physicians across the world. And the AAD says that, unless the skin is actually dirty, it's not necessary to bathe children any more than once or twice a week.

That's extraordinary. Think about the level of evidence required for the organization to make a statement like that. It's quite courageous, too. Many dermatologists have relationships with skincare companies. Some of these companies sell soap, and they're likely to see their sales go down as a result of such a recommendation. But despite the pushback that the AAD members might get from skincare companies, the doctors' group felt the scientific evidence was so strong that it needed to make a stand.

Now listen: If your kid is dirty—if he or she has been playing out in the mud all day, or with worms or frogs or any of the billion other things kids do to dirty up their bodies—then go ahead and give your child a bath. The same thing applies if the child is sweaty, or has body odour—as the AAD points out.

Some parents will shudder at the thought of bathing their children just once or twice every seven days. Going from a bath a day to a bath a week seems like quite a change. One way to start is to simply avoid using soap and cleanser. Give your kids a quick shower or bath and let the water drain over them.

Just remember that the reflex to begin that evening ritual, to get your kids in the bath or shower and scrub them every single night . . . is too much. Not only do children not need it, but it may actually be harmful for the skin. You're likely increasing their risk of developing eczema or other atopic conditions, or developing an allergy to a product ingredient. You may also be altering the delicate balance of the skin's microbiome.

The AAD issued the guidelines for children aged 6 to 11. I think they should apply to those between the ages of two and puberty. In fact, I don't use soap at all in my house; I use only synthetic cleansers with little to no allergens and irritants. I would suggest the same products for children that I've suggested for adults—the ones I listed in Chapter 6.

Of course, I still recommend following healthy handwashing practices, including washing hands before meals and after trips to the washroom, to minimize the spread of communicable diseases.

Teens

Things change after puberty: I get it. As I write this, all three of my boys are adolescents. The AAD has different advice for young people who've become teenagers. It suggests that they bathe daily, and wash their faces every morning and evening.

I don't think an all-over washing is required every day with cleansers. A daily rinse, maybe, and then use cleansers in places where oil can begin to be an issue, like trunks. Also use cleansers on odiferous areas like underarms, groins and feet.

The big problem for teenagers is acne. When my older sons started to get some acne I brought home the foaming facial wash I'd created myself, which is called FormulaB, after my eldest boy, Brandon. The acne wash doesn't have any fragrance, parabens or formaldehyde preservatives. Nor does it have problematic detergents like sodium lauryl sulphate or cocamidopropyl betaine.

What I discovered, though, is that my boys didn't know what to do with it. They slathered it on their faces as if it was moisturizer and then tried to rinse it off. There was no lathering action involved. It was funny—what a fail for a dermatologist! I guess I'd never shown my kids how to wash their faces.

In slight contrast to the AAD's advice, I'd suggest that teenagers wash their faces only at night with a cleanser. You can certainly rinse anytime. Young men or women who are on medication for acne may find that many facial cleansers are too harsh for skin that's been dried out by what their doctor has prescribed them. In that case, I'd try using a non-foaming, lipid-free cleanser or a micellar cleanser. If you want something a little stronger, use the two products together.

For those who are starting to put on makeup, I'd suggest going with options that are oil-free. If you do choose to use cover-up, find something that's oil-free as well. Mineral- and powder-based makeups are good for oily, acne-prone skin. Avoid the makeups that include salicylic acid as a therapy for acne. Your makeup should be your makeup. Don't combine acne medicine and makeup. Rather, wear makeup during the day and acne medicine at night.

As for products, I really do suggest the same products for teens as I do for adults, so consult the lists in Chapter 6. If you have acne, opt for a foaming facial cleanser without the bells and whistles—that is, without fragrances and cool-sounding organics. The ones from Cetaphil, CeraVe and Toleriane are great, as is Neutrogena's foaming facial cleanse and my own formulation, FormulaB cleanse.

Finally, teens who are acne prone need to watch what sorts of sunscreen they use. In my experience, sunscreen can aggravate acne. For acne-prone faces, the lighter, fluid sunscreen is better because it's less likely to cause breakouts. I'd suggest that teens consider using the following products:

- Clinique SPF 50 Mineral Fluid for Face
- La Roche-Posay Anthelios Ultra Light Sunscreen Fluid SPF 60
- Neutrogena Clear Face Sunscreen Lotion SPF 60
- Neutrogena Pure & Free Liquid Sunscreen SPF 50

We're apt to treat kids as though they're fragile things who need to be washed and scrubbed and showered and all the rest, every day. Just remember, the scientific evidence suggests that such practices are doing more harm than good. Exposure to the great wide world is good for kids—in terms of cleanliness, as well as life.

Minimalist Skincare: Fighting Aging, Preserving Skin Health and Enhancing Beauty

One of the more fascinating recent trends in the beauty product market is Korean skincare. Borrowing the logic of its name from the "K-pop" of the Seoul singer Psy's "Gangnam Style," the mania for "K-Beauty" is such that the makeup retailer Sephora created an online mini-store that specializes in products from the Asian nation, with names like Dr. Jart+ and AmorePacific.

The epitome of this grooming and hygiene obsession is the 10-step Korean beauty routine, which got its start in Seoul's Gangnam District. The routine begins with the application of makeup-removing towelettes and progresses through three types of cleanses, then exfoliation and toner, followed by the application of essence and ampoules, a facial mask and eye cream, emulsifier and, finally, the 10th step, a rich moisturizing sleep pack—all in the name of age-defying, healthy skin. The whole thing requires about 45 minutes to run through.

Meanwhile, in this dermatologist's opinion, the women pursuing the Korean skincare regimen would be a lot better off if they just used a non-foaming cleanser and invested the rest of that time in some beauty sleep.

Then there's the other extreme: doing nothing. Like, *absolutely* nothing. A thriving subculture of people who subscribe to a do-nothing skincare philosophy exists on the Internet. Representative of it is Robert Brumm, a 42-year-old Wisconsin writer who decided one day to stop washing with soap. He's also sworn off shampoo. You might think that today he sits in a garbage can, warding people off with his smell. He wondered that himself when he started out. And actually, things started out pretty tough. "Most of it in the early parts is psychological," Brumm told me when I spoke to him. "You just feel kind of gross. You have it drilled into your brain, 'You're not clean without soap.'" The first day or two went by and Brumm felt dirty. Greasy. Unkempt. As though a thin layer of invisible oil covered every bit of his body.

His wife didn't mind much. What troubled her at first was Brumm's new smell. She'd been used to the odour of his shampoo. "You just don't smell like Rob," she said when she gave him a hug one day.

It's important to know at this point that Brumm would take showers. He'd get in there and allow the water to sluice over his skin. The thing he *didn't* do was pick up the soap. He just let it sit there on its dish in the little recess in the shower. He didn't wash his hair, either. There was that short time soon after he stopped washing that his skin felt oily. Then one day, a few weeks later, he stepped from the shower, towelled off and just felt normal. Not only that: "I started noticing my skin was a lot softer and it didn't dry out," Brumm said. "And my face wasn't breaking out as often." His hair improved, too. It looked greasier than normal for a while, but then that normalized and his hair looked just like it always had.

After two months of soapless showering (he did wash his hands after toilet trips), you might think Brumm was so smelly that people would avoid him on public transit and his wife would have banished him to the guest bedroom. But that wasn't the case at all. Remember, Brumm still *showered*. He allowed water to go over his skin and get rid of the sweat and anything else his skin had been exposed to that day. In fact, he smelled fine. He *felt* fine, too. If anything, his skin was healthier and less blemish-ridden than it had been before he started this experiment. His wife's used to it now, too. "You just smell like you," she tells him.

Brumm's not the only one to attempt this. The do-nothing crowd reject the precepts of the contemporary beauty industry, the "more is more" ethos, trading in the cleansers and emulsifiers and everything else to espouse a minimalist beauty regimen. Sometimes they call it the "paleo skincare" movement, because they're presumably pursuing beauty tactics similar to those in Paleolithic times. Others, who have simply stopped washing their hair with shampoo, say they've embraced the "no poo" lifestyle (for "no shampoo").

I haven't done either of those things, nor do I recommend them. I'm not as hardcore as the paleo and other bloggers who swear off shampoo and dispense with using any products whatsoever. I *do* have a beauty regimen—but rather than subscribing to paleo skincare, I try to stay away from any ideology at all. Instead, I sub- scribe to an approach that may predate even Paleolithic times. It's called "common sense."

Here's how it works: I limit myself to the beauty rituals that have been proven by science to lead to healthy skin that slows the signs of aging. Notice that I say *slow* rather than reverse. Because I don't think you can actually *reverse* aging. At least, not through dermatological means. Not with creams or anything topical. You can reverse aging for a time with cosmetic surgery—and for that, you need a great plastic surgeon. But I don't think you need to see a plastic surgeon to have great skin throughout your life. A whole series of things have

been shown to fight aging and care for the skin in a healthy and
natural manner. Not all are natural or organic. And I use them.
Science has given us some remarkable things over the years,
including electric cars, robot vacuum cleaners and fans that don't
have any blades. As well as some synthetic molecules that happen to
slow the signs of aging. I'm not going to avoid using those just
because they don't come from Mother Nature. Nope—I'm going to
use everything I can to look great and healthy for as long as possible.
Here, then, is my step-by-step regimen designed to do just that.

Common-Sense Beauty

First of all, let me break it down for you. Aging is 60 percent genetics. Whether your parents had good skin, whether they looked
good into their sixties, seventies and eighties—a lot of that is luck.
Some of the reasons for that have to do with the DNA you inherit.
At this point in medical history you can't change your genetic
makeup—although it's possible that you may be able to do something about it in the future. (See Chapter 10 for more about that.)

At this point, you can affect about 40 percent of the aging
process. Whether you bake yourself in the sun—that affects things.
Same with whether you smoke. And then come the things that
might surprise you. People tend not to consider what you eat, the
quality of your sleep and your decision to exercise as important
factors in a beauty regimen. But they are. In this chapter I'm going
to tell you every tactic I know that has been scientifically proven to
affect the rate at which skin ages. Let's get started.

Exercise

There's a good reason why I have a trainer over to my house at 7 a.m.
several times a week. Exercise is really great for the skin. You can see

it in the healthy, fit people you know. And it turns out there's something to the science behind it. In 2014, Mark Tarnopolsky of McMaster University conducted a study that looked into the relationship between skin, aging and exercise. Tarnopolsky was already well known for experiments he'd conducted with mice that had been bred to age faster than normal mice. He'd shown that the progress of time slowed for these fast-aging mice if they did one thing: exercise regularly.

That's right: These unusual mice, genetically engineered to age faster than normal, tended to develop wrinkled skin and greying fur a lot faster than ordinary mice.

Unless they exercised.

If the mice exercised, their fur didn't go grey and their skin didn't get wrinkly. They just looked like normal mice. Would exercise have a similar effect in humans? Tarnopolsky was intrigued enough by the results that he created an experiment to find out. He gathered 29 people who ranged from 20 to 84 years old. Half of them were regular exercisers, with three or more bouts of physical activity a week; the other half didn't exercise regularly. Then Tarnopolsky had their skin analyzed. The results were about what he would have expected—with one caveat. In general, the older the people, the thinner their stratum corneum and the less elastic their dermis. Except in those who exercised regularly. Once they started getting past the age of 40, the exercisers had significantly younger skin. Exercisers who were in their sixties had dermal thickness similar to people in their twenties.

Could the exercise have slowed the skin's aging? Tarnopolsky wanted to investigate further. It was possible, after all, that something else was causing the better skin. Diet. Type of shoe worn. Lots of different causes were possible. So he did another test. He took some of the people over the age of 65 who didn't exercise, and conducted another experiment on them. First he took a sample of their skin. Then he put them on an exercise program. A relatively simple and achievable one—one that required them to conduct aerobic exercise for 30 minutes twice a week.

After three months of exercise, Tarnopolsky took another skin sample from his (now considerably more fit) subjects. Analysis showed that the subjects' skin had changed dramatically. Their stratum corneum and dermis were so different that they seemed to have shed several decades of aging. The people who once had skin typical of seniors now better resembled people who were between 20 and 40 years old. "It was pretty remarkable to see," Tarnopolsky told *The New York Times*.

Bear in mind that the skin they sampled came from people's buttocks, because Tarnopolsky wanted to insulate against the results being affected by sun exposure.

Would something similar happen for the face? I'm not saying three months of exercise is going to remove 25 years from your face. That doesn't happen for everyone. Nor am I going to recommend a certain type of exercise as having better wrinkle-fighting properties than any other. The science just isn't there yet. But what I am going to do is recommend that you engage in *some* type of exercise. Physical activity on a regular basis will make your skin look better, particularly for people who are getting fit for their first time. So—if you're looking for a low-cost, age-defying beauty regimen that actually works, try exercise.

Airborne Pollutants

Dermatologists like me have spent the last 20 years talking about how harmful ultraviolet exposure can be for the skin. The public seems to have received that message—and just in case you haven't, I'll provide my specific recommendations for sunscreen later in this chapter. For now, I want to discuss something that dermatologists may be discussing for the *next* 20 years: airborne pollutants.

Automobiles, wood fires, general industry and solvent

manufacturing and use are among the factors responsible for the many foreign substances in the air. They have names like particulate matter, volatile organic compounds, nitrogen oxide, ozone and polycyclic aromatic hydrocarbons. A spate of recent dermatological research looked at the aging effect of traffic fumes and other airborne chemicals. Turns out it's extensive.

Scientists have found that places with higher levels of air pollution tend to have greater amounts of skin eruptions due to factors like atopic dermatitis. A lot of these substances also look like they're encouraging skin aging. Maybe they're promoting factors that trigger the development of pigment spots, also known as liver spots. Nanoscale particulate matter, which can be anything from microscopic metal fragments to organic compounds, can be particularly reactive with the skin, contributing to inflammation as well as wrinkles and the loss of skin elasticity.

One of the world's experts on the effect of air pollution on skin aging is Professor Jean Krutmann, director of the Leibniz Research Institute for Environmental Medicine in Germany. He recently conducted a study in Germany and China that examined whether cheek age spots correlated with increases in atmospheric nitrogen dioxide, approximately 80 percent of which comes from automobile exhaust. Remarkably, just 10 micrograms of NO_2 correlated with an increase in cheek age spots of 25 percent. (Major metropolitan areas around the world regularly see atmospheric levels of NO_2 surpass 200 micrograms, particularly in summer.)

"It is not a problem that is limited to China or India," Krutmann told *The Guardian* newspaper in a recent article. "We have it in Paris, in London, wherever you have larger urban agglomerations you have it."

U.K. cosmetic doctor Mervyn Patterson calls traffic pollution "the single most toxic substance for skin." His theory, according to *The Guardian*, is that the reactive air-pollution agents trigger skin-inflammation pathways, which in turn activate melanocytes, the

pigment factories that create sun spots. "Other pathways ignite
messengers that make blood vessels grow, that's what results in
increased redness and potentially rosacea," Patterson said. "Also, if
you damage skin, it goes into repair mode and excites enzymes
which re-absorb damaged collagen. When you have too much
chronic inflammation, these enzymes remove more collagen than
your skin can create. This produces skin laxity and that's where fine
lines and wrinkles come in."

What to do? I mean, we can't all just hide out in North Dakota
our entire lives. One predictable response would be to go home each
night, whip out the most abrasive and soapiest of face scrubs and
attempt to sandblast those pollutants off the skin. Unfortunately, that
would turn out to be one of the worst things you could do, according
to Patterson—and I concur. The reason, of course, happens to be
this book's central argument: that such interventions damage the
skin's innate barrier function and impede the body's natural
protective mechanism. "The skin is trying its damnedest to make
this wonderful defence mechanism," Patterson told *The Guardian.*
"And what do women and men do? They scrub the hell out of it. It
just doesn't make sense."

So how to protect against air pollution? One method is to use
mineral makeup. Minerals like titanium and zinc help block out
pollutants. I like to use a tinted titanium sunblock, like Chantecaille
Just Skin Tinted Moisturizer or La Roche-Posay Mineral SPF 50.
The Chantecaille has some botanicals in it; at around $100, it's also
not cheap. But it works for me, and I've used it for more than 10 years
without a reaction. There are lots of tinted titanium screens out there.
They create a barrier that doesn't allow nitrogen oxide, or much of
anything else, to get past it to damage the skin. If you do opt to go that
route, remember to cleanse the facial skin each night.

One more thing. Air pollution that's harmful to the skin doesn't
just come from diesel exhaust and factories. Another source is

cigarette smoke, which ages your skin and is harmful to your body in many other ways. In fact, I'd argue that few other human behaviours age your skin as effectively as smoking. If you want to look like a wraith at age 40, and even worse by age 60, then smoke. Inhale nicotine and various other pollutants into your chest. Exhale it out. Repeat many times per day. For the rest of us? If you want age-defying skin, avoid cigarette smoke, and those who exhale it, as much as possible.

DO CLAY MASKS HELP THE SKIN?

People ask me about clay masks all the time. To put it at its most basic, clay is an old-fashioned way to suck out the stuff that gets clogged in your pores. You slather on the mud, it dries, and as it dries it pulls out whatever's clogging you. I'd say that most people don't need clay masks. But if you have a lot of clogged pores, they can help.

Diet

For many decades, conventional wisdom held that diet didn't have any effect on human dermatology. What you put into your mouth was not supposed to affect the skin. Today, we know that's just plain wrong. Diet can affect the skin in numerous different ways.

Let's talk about aging first. A major factor in aging is the status of the skin's collagen and elastic fibres, which tend to undergo a process called glycation as you get older. In glycation, connections known as covalent bonds are established between amino acids located in collagen and elastic fibres in the dermis, the skin's underlayer. The more glycation, the more connections there are between the fibres in the skin, and the less the skin is able to spring back into place. Robbed of its youthful elasticity, glycated skin looks saggy and stiff, and it wrinkles more.

The process of glycation is happening all the time in the human body. Science hasn't figured out a way to detach the bonds forming between all those collagen and elastin fibres. We *can* slow down the process, however. And one way to do that is by changing one's diet. Foods that have been grilled, fried or roasted—i.e., a lot of what we eat—tend to promote glycation, so increasing the proportion of raw foods in your diet seems like a good bet. (Some herbs and spices, such as oregano, cinnamon, cloves, ginger and garlic, may inhibit glycation, but the science seems weak here.) According to Rajani Katta and Samir Desai, dermatology faculty at Baylor College of Medicine, curtailing the body's production of glucose and fructose is an important way to curtail glycation. And to do that, you pursue a low-glycemic diet. Basically, you eat like a diabetic. Eat foods that don't have much sugar in them and that are low in carbs. Avoid chocolate, quit those milkshakes, put away those jujubes. Trade white bread and white rice for whole grains and brown rice.

This also turns out to be the advice for how to limit acne, another skin malady that dermatologists have realized can be influenced by diet. The science is a lot better established here. For example, several randomized controlled trials associated low-glycemic-index diets with a decreased incidence of acne. Avoiding dairy products that may contain growth hormones may also help decrease acne.

Then there's the most common form of cancer in the United States: nonmelanoma skin cancer. The likelihood of developing it can be decreased with some key changes to the usual Western diet. The science is good here, too. Back in the 1970s, researchers found that skin cancer developed in only 7 percent of UVA-irradiated mice fed a diet rich in vitamins C and E and glutathione. In UVA-irradiated mice that pursued a regular diet, 30 percent developed the cancer. Other substances that have a prophylactic effect on the development of skin cancer include beta carotene, selenium, and such

phytonutrients as curcumin, lycopene and genistein. Also, antioxidants like resveratrol (found in grapes) and ellagic acid (in raspber-
ries) tend to mop up the free radicals known to promote cancer.

You might be tempted to act on this information by taking
supplements rich in antioxidants and phytonutrients. But for
whatever reason, such tactics don't seem to have much of an effect
on skin cancer risk. More bad news is the fact that the typical
Western diet of hamburgers, pizzas and extra-whip grande mochas
seems to be really bad for the skin. Rather, the better strategy is to
pursue the same plant-based, whole-food diet that many doctors
recommend for reducing the risk of everything from cardiovascular
disease to diabetes. "It is possible to eat your way to healthy skin,"
says Zoe Draelos, a North Carolina–based dermatologist whom I
cited earlier in the book and who's written about the interaction of
diet and skin. In particular, Katta and Desai suggest the DASH diet
(Dietary Approaches to Stop Hypertension). Originally designed
to curtail high blood pressure, it contains enough plants and whole
foods to also help the skin. Avoid foods that have been fried, grilled
and roasted. And limit that sugar!

Beauty Products That Actually Work

The product recommendations that follow assume that you're not
currently dealing with sensitive skin. You already know that I think
many products aren't necessary and that most people who have
sensitive skin can deal with the problem by following the product-
elimination process I described in Chapter 6. Once their sensitive
skin has settled, my patients tend to be very happy that their skin is
quiet—and then the next question comes: What can I use?
Typically, my patients want some anti-aging stuff. Or a cream that
smells nice. Or they say: I miss my shampoo. Even if you've had

sensitive skin, experienced reactions to cosmetics, or are suffering from one of the commonly associated skin conditions, you can try various things. Once you're better and not reactive, you can try whatever you like. You just have to understand the dos and don'ts.

When choosing your products, remember that it's not about the newest or greatest, or even, for that matter, the most expensive. You can get very good skincare for very little money. What it *is* about is which products have the best science to back them up.

People are always coming into the office and asking me, What's the best cleanser? The best sunscreen? The absolutely most wonderful moisturizer? It's the most common question in any dermatological office, and it drives dermatologists like me a little crazy. Because these patients are asking *the wrong question.* A single best *anything* doesn't exist. Different people have different needs.

The right question is, What's the best _____ *for me.* The best thing for your friend is not the best thing for you. Do you have acne or rosacea? Are you fair? What's your ethnicity? Ethnicity and the amount of sun damage you have is a bigger issue than your age. The skin of an older person is different, but the recommendations are the same. The major difference between old and young skin is usually the extent of sun exposure.

One final word: So much of skin and hair care is based on psychology. Some patients feel their product works better if it costs more. That's bunk.

If you really want to attack your aging head-on, see a dermatologist. Products are only going to do so much. Topical products will slow the clock. They won't turn it back. If you want to actually reverse your aging, you'll need sit down and think seriously about whether you want to conduct a more radical intervention, such as filler, injections like Botox or plastic surgery. Each one comes with its own risks, which we don't discuss here. With the right professional, they can be effective.

Cleansers

For all my ranting about not washing, it is necessary to cleanse the face of makeup and pollution. But unless you were out all night hunting, you don't need to do this in the morning. Do it in the evening, before you go to bed. A *perfect* method for cleansing the face and body does not exist. Many cleansers contain fragrance—and by now, you know how I feel about fragrance. You also know that I, like many dermatologists, believe that soap should not be used for cleansing the face, and that we should limit the use of soap on the body.

Thankfully, manufacturers have realized that soap is detrimental to the skin and have made an effort to make newer cleansers with synthetic or even plant-based surfactants that don't strip the skin's natural oils and are close to its natural pH.

My ideal cleanser product recommendations for the face and body are much the same as what I suggested for the middle phase of the product-elimination diet—low to no foaming, fragrance-free and low-allergenic.

NON-FOAMING FACIAL CLEANSERS

- Avène Tolérance Extrême Cleansing Lotion
- CeraVe Hydrating Cleanser
- Cetaphil Gentle Skin Cleanser
- La Roche-Posay Toleriane Dermo-Cleanser
- Neutrogena Ultra Gentle Hydrating Cleanser
- Spectro Derm Cleanser for Dry Skin (not Spectro Jel, which contains a formaldehyde-releasing preservative)

FOAMING FACIAL CLEANSERS

- CeraVe Foaming Facial Cleanser
- Cetaphil Foaming Facial Wash
- FormulaB Cleanse soap-free mildly foaming cleanser
- La Roche-Posay Toleriane Purifying Foaming Cream

The problem, as I've mentioned before, is that some people don't like the lipid-free cleansers or non-foaming cleansers. "They're too gentle," some say. "I don't feel like they're cleaning my skin." Others dislike the fact that such cleansers don't create suds. If you really don't like the gentle cleansers and feel as though you simply must return to more traditional products, please opt for something that minimizes the use of added fragrances or allergenic botanicals. Bear in mind that the more foam the cleanser creates, the more irritating and drying it usually is for your skin. Some patients with oily, acne-prone skin may benefit from using such higher-foaming cleansers. However, they're the first thing I stop in patients with sensitive or reactive skin. Also try to avoid colouring agents. Finally, try to keep all other aspects of your beauty regimen the same when you introduce a higher-foaming cleanser, so that if your skin *does* react to the new product, at least you'll know the cause.

Another option? The fashion magazines and online forums have been extolling the virtues of *double cleansing*. Brands from Dermalogica to Super Facialist are offering *pre-cleanse* products—wipes and oils designed to be used *before* your usual cleanser. These products have arisen because some people think non-foaming cleansers may not remove all your makeup. I hesitate to tell patients to pre-cleanse their skin at night to remove anything. But if you must, then consider using a micellar water cleanser after you wash with a non-foaming cleanser. You'll need an absorbent cotton pad to apply the cleanser. Use micellar water first, then wash with the non-foaming cleanser, or vice versa. I like:

- Bioderma Sensibio H2O Micelle Solution
- Reversa Cleansing Micellar Solution

Some patients are intent on using natural alternatives. My concern with some of these natural products is that they're often loaded with botanicals, which add little to their usefulness while increasing the likelihood of triggering a skin reaction. But if your skin is not reactive, and you're not suffering from eczema or some other skin condition, then go ahead and try what you like. I'd suggest:

- Dr. Roebuck's Cleanse Natural Nourishing Crème Cleanser: I've used this myself, and quite liked it. Bear in mind that it contains some botanicals from the Asteraceae family, which can be allergenic.
- Mother Dirt Cleanser: From AOBiome, this mild and gentle foaming cleanser with a texture like shaving cream is designed to preserve the skin's microbiome.

BODY CLEANSERS

1. Syndet bars: The syndet bars, or beauty bars, will make you feel cleaner, as they have some soap in them.
   - Aveeno Moisturizing Bar
   - CeraVe Hydrating Cleansing Bar
   - Cetaphil Gentle Cleansing Bar (has masking fragrance)
   - Dove Sensitive Skin Beauty Bar (contains the allergen CAPB)
2. Body washes: Remember, only wash your bits—underarms, groin and feet—unless you've been rolling around in the dirt!
   - Cetaphil Restoraderm Body Wash
   - Exederm Cleansing Body Wash
   - La Roche-Posay Lipikar Syndet Cleansing Body Cream-Gel (contains SLS and foams)
   - Skinfix Soothing Wash (does contain some botanicals and several allergens, but a good option for patients who want more naturals)

SHOULD I USE A CLARISONIC OR ANY OTHER
SKINCARE FACE BRUSH?

The Clarisonic skincare face brush is not principally designed to be abrasive to the skin or to have an exfoliating effect—although some minor exfoliation likely does occur. Rather, its oscillating action, analogous to a massage, is designed to increase blood flow to the skin. The face brushes can be expensive, and while I don't think they're necessary, there is some science showing that such products are able to increase the penetration rate of ingredients like Retin-A, retinol and vitamin C. This in turn suggests that, by using a Clarisonic, you can get away with using a lower-concentration (and less irritating) version of your skincare products—which would turn out to be cheaper in the long run. For example, rather than using a more expensive 10 percent concentration of vitamin C, you could opt for a more reasonably priced 5 percent of vitamin C—then use the Clarisonic in the hope that the device increases the vitamin C actually penetrating the skin.

Sunscreens

When I was a resident training to become a dermatologist, I had an elderly professor who became quite perplexed when female patients would ask him about anti-wrinkle creams. His standard answer was "Go home and look at your backside—sunscreen is all you need." His answer might have been rude, but he also had a point. The parts of our bodies not exposed to the sun don't get as many wrinkles as the ones that are, a reflection of the fact that UV radiation is the single biggest contributor to aging skin—thicker and saggier skin, wrinkles and brown pigmentation.

Consequently, the most effective way to prevent skin aging is sunscreen. So what makes a good sunscreen? Well, lots of things. Sunscreens need to protect against both wavelengths of ultraviolet light, known as UVA and UVB, which have been associated with skin cancer and skin aging. They need to be stable both in the bottle and on the skin. They should minimize unnecessary extra ingredients, such as fragrance molecules. And when possible, they should also feature an opaque substance like titanium or zinc that helps physically block the sun's rays from reaching the skin and protect it from longer UVA light.

In 2012, thanks to consumer confusion about the meaning behind SPF, regulators from both the Canadian and American governments changed the guidelines for indicating sunscreen effectiveness. It all has to do with the term SPF, which stands for sun-protection factor. To assess a given product's SPF level, two milligrams of sunscreen is applied per square centimetre of skin. (That's really slathering it on. It amounts to applying an entire teaspoon to each of your major body parts—a teaspoon for each arm, for the face, and even more for the larger areas, like the chest and legs. Few consumers would ever use that much sunscreen.) Then solar radiation is applied to a volunteer's skin to see how long that skin takes to burn. Based on the result, the product is assigned an SPF rating. If a volunteer patient burns in 10 minutes, the application of an SPF 15 sunscreen will lengthen the time to burning by a factor of 15, so the subject would be able to stay in the sun for 150 minutes without burning.

Here's the thing, though: The test measures only the extent to which the sunscreen protects against the rays that actually cause a visible burn on your skin—the UVB rays. SPF gives absolutely no indication of the extent to which the product protects your skin from UVA rays. That's important because UVA rays are the major contributor to skin cancer and skin aging. Which makes the whole sunscreen rating system kind of silly, right? Most of us are wearing the sunscreen to prevent cancer and skin aging. And yet the product's key measure of effectiveness says nothing about the extent to which a given product protects us from that! Nor do the regulators have any plans to change the situation, mostly because it's difficult to measure UVA damage.

Which brings us back to the labelling changes. Before 2012, the regulations did a poor job of assessing a given sunscreen's UVA-ray protection. Since then, only sunscreens that protect you against UVA rays are allowed to call themselves "broad spectrum" sunscreens. They may also say something like "Protects against both UVA and UVB rays." However, consumers still didn't have any indication how much UVA protection the products include.

Until recently. In an effort to help consumers know whether the UVA protection is adequate, the skincare industry worked with the EU and decided the following: If the UVA symbol on the sunscreen bottle has a circle on it, the UVA protection is at least a third of the overall SPF rating. It means the sunscreen is a good one.

Still, the evaluations in Canada assess only the first hour of a sunscreen's effectiveness. So keep in mind that the sunscreen's protection may not last all that long.

Thanks to all this confusion, I recommend only sunscreens from companies that are transparent in their scientific research, so that I can assess how much the product protects against UVA—as well as the product's photostability. For these reasons, I tend to favour sunscreens from these companies:

- Avène
- Bioderma
- La Roche-Posay
- Neutrogena
- Ombrelle
- Vichy

Another sunscreen-related question I get involves the value of the SPF rating. Is higher better? The short answer is yes. The longer answer is, higher is better only up to a point. It all comes back to that SPF test again. Say you're a company testing a sunscreen that contains three ingredients that absorb UVB. Your SPF lab test on volunteers gives you an SPF of 20—at first.

But then in an effort to make your sunscreen better, you decide you need to add sunscreen ingredients that absorb or block UVA. So you add two extra ingredients, do the lab test again, and come out with a much higher number—because the substances you added to block UVA rays work against UVB rays, too.

Sunscreen X = 3 UVB ingredients = SPF 20
Sunscreen X = 3 UVB ingredients + 2 UVA ingredients = SPF 80

The problem is, things get tricky after 50. A 50-rated SPF blocks 98 percent of UVB rays. Higher than 50 and the benefits become incrementally smaller. There's a false security to them. Someone might think they're okay to stay out in the full sun for hours on end—because the sunscreen is blocking the burn-causing UVB rays. But what the person is really doing is exposing him- or herself to wrinkle- and cancer-causing UVA rays. To reduce the risks, the United States, the European Union and Australia, among others, are limiting the upper range of SPF numbers to a 50+ rating because SPF is a limiting test for the full measure of sunscreen efficacy.

Armed with all this information, what do you do? I suggest you choose a product rated SPF 30 or higher from one of my suggested companies—particularly when you're out in the sun during peak UV-index hours of 11 a.m. to 3 p.m. And bonus points if you use a product that features a circled UVA symbol.

WHAT ABOUT SUNSCREENS IN MOISTURIZERS AND MAKEUP?
I used to discourage my patients from using moisturizers or makeup that also featured sunscreen. Sunscreens are sunscreens, I would say,

and moisturizers are moisturizers. If you want a good sunscreen, use a sunscreen.

My reason involves the way sunscreens are rated. Remember that the SPF tests require the application of two milligrams per square centimetre of skin. That's a lot of sunscreen. Would you apply a teaspoon of foundation to your face? No! So in the morning, when you apply your usual pea-sized amount of foundation that has an SPF of 15, you might be getting an SPF of only 5. If you're lucky. Also—most makeups and moisturizers don't have good UVA protectants in them.

Having said all that, I've grown mellower over the decades I've practised. The most important thing about sunscreen is that patients use it. If you're realistically going to use only a single product—say, facial foundation—then it's better for that product to include sunscreen. Even if you're only getting an SPF of 5.

SHOULD I WEAR SUNSCREEN YEAR ROUND?

The short answer is yes. The most important study looking at sunscreen and skin cancer prevention was conducted in Australia. It showed that over a 10-year time period, the people who used sunscreen every day had significantly lower rates of melanoma and squamous-cell carcinoma skin cancer. Those who are concerned about their looks will also be interested to learn that sunscreen substantially decreased wrinkles and other signs of skin aging.

Yet the study took place in *Australia*. Where many places are sunny all the time. I hesitate to say this because consistent sunscreen use is really important. But let's be realistic. I live in Toronto, where the winters can stick around for five months. If I go outside for a walk or to ski, I wear a chemical sunscreen from one of my recommended companies. On the days I'm not outside much? I think it's fine to wear a tinted physical sunscreen product like La Roche-Posay Anthelios Mineral Tinted Ultra-Fluid Lotion SPF 50 or SkinCeuticals Physical Fusion UV Defense. And as I suggested in my answer to the preceding question, I'm even growing comfortable with my patients using foundations with physical sun blockers like titanium or zinc. They're fine protection in the dark winter months, since they reduce incidental UV rays, and, because they provide a physical barrier, they also increase pollution protection. Just remember, when you're out in peak sun, use the best science has to offer.

WILL THE CHEMICALS IN SUNSCREEN IRRITATE MY SKIN?

It's a question I get asked a lot. Patients worry about the absorption of sunscreen's active chemicals, and wonder whether they should use sunscreens that employ physical blockers, like zinc and titanium.

I get it—although I do point out that zinc and titanium are chemicals, too. Then I get to the pertinent discussion. Sunscreens employ chemicals with names like benzophenone, Parsal 1789 or Mexoryl. The substances are absorbed into the skin, where they react with UV radiation, in turn preventing the radiation from acting on the skin.

In contrast, physical-blocking sunscreens that employ zinc and titanium work mostly by *reflecting* UV light. These sunscreens do protect against UVB and UVA, but they're not the best technology available. I generally try to steer people to the chemical sunscreens. But if you're really concerned, then the physical-block sunscreens I prefer are:

- Avène Mineral Cream SPF 50+
- Avène Mineral High Protection Tinted Compact SPF 50
- Bioderma Photoderm Compact Mineral SPF 50+
- EltaMD UV Physical Broad-Spectrum SPF 41
- La Roche-Posay Anthelios Mineral Tinted Ultra-Fluid Lotion SPF 50

- Neutrogena Sheer Zinc Lotion SPF 50
- SkinCeuticals Physical Fusion UV Defense SPF 50

Sometimes when people use sunscreen they experience a burning or stinging sensation. That's usually not an allergic reaction. Allergy to sunscreens does happen, but the incidence is low. The most common offenders are benzophenone and Parsal 1789. If you have sensitive, reactive or eczematous skin, physical sunscreen may be easier to use, particularly on the face.

Moisturizers

When it comes to moisturizers, the drugstores, beauty counters and online merchants feature a bewildering array of choices—numbering in the thousands. There is no single best miracle moisturizing cream. Instead, there are really good ingredients. The rest is personal choice and price point. So what are the ingredients that make a good moisturizer? And then, as many of my patients wonder: Are there any moisturizers that have been proven to reduce the signs of aging?

When asked such questions, dermatologists like to look at the science. And for moisturizers, this is challenging. One of the age-old tricks in the cosmetic industry is reduction of wrinkles with a moisturizer. A moisturizer will immediately reduce the appearance of fine lines by about 15 percent—but not permanently. The wrinkles will return once the skin dries out. Rather than removing wrinkles, a moisturizer does what its name suggests—it helps restore the skin's natural barrier. There's not a lot of science to show that moisturizers reduce the signs of skin aging over time. And the studies that *have* indicated age-defying benefits tend to be backed by cosmetic companies, which means their results are suspect. Companies tend to be more aggressive with their claims about cosmeceuticals, which fall somewhere between cosmetics and drugs. In fact, cosmeceuticals for skin rejuvenation and anti-aging are the fastest-growing segment of the skincare market. And yet most of these products lack good clinical trials to substantiate their efficacy.

The easier way to think about choosing a skincare product that goes beyond moisturizing is to consider what the skin actually requires. In order to be healthy and efficiently slow the aging process, the skin needs:

1. Protection from the sun
2. Maintenance of its barrier function (moisturizing)
3. Reduction of oxidative stress on the skin
4. Cell signallers, which fight the signs of aging by boosting turnover of skin cells and collagen production
5. Exfoliation of the dead uppermost skin cells

The first item gets handled by sunscreen. Items three to five we'll cover later in the chapter. For now, we'll talk about item two—maintenance of the skin's barrier function. This task is carried out by your basic moisturizer with no added anti-aging or rejuvenation ingredients. Our skin barrier is under constant assault. By soap, by sun, by particulate matter and air pollution. Also by oxidative decay—meaning the natural aging process, in which oxygen free radicals damage the integral parts of the skin matrix, among them cellular proteins, cell membranes, enzymes, DNA and RNA.

One effect of all these assaults is that the skin's brick-and-mortar matrix gets damaged. This leads to the evaporation of water from the skin, a phenomenon called transepidermal water loss, or TEWL, which causes dryness, cracking and all sorts of dermatological conditions. The extent of TEWL provides scientists with an objective measure of skin health. Unhealthy skin tends to feature lots of it.

The ingredients that cosmetic companies use in moisturizers fall into three broad categories. The first is *occlusives*: substances that block water molecules from evaporating off the outermost layer of the stratum corneum. Since these substances tend to be thick and goopy, they can be difficult to actually rub into the dermis. The most effective occlusive is petroleum jelly, followed by lanolin, mineral oil and such silicones as dimethicone.

The second category of moisturizers is *humectants*. When applied to the skin, humectants attract water. They're supposed to improve hydration of the stratum corneum. But what they can end up doing is attracting *transepidermal* water rather than atmospheric water. The effect? Humectants actually can pull water *out* of the skin, which can exacerbate the very dryness they're supposed to address. Humectants include glycerine, sorbitol, urea and such alpha hydroxy acids as lactic or glycolic acids.

Then come the *emollients*, which have occlusive properties because they block moisture from evaporating off the skin. But they also have a smoothing function, which they achieve by filling the matrix with oil molecules. Sometimes emollients have vitamins added to them, such as vitamins A, D or E, but according to researchers, scientific studies have failed to demonstrate that these vitamins have any effect on the skin. Mineral oil, lanolin, cholesterol, squalene and structural lipids are all considered to be emollients, as are palm oil and coconut oil.

One strategy cosmetic companies use when constructing moisturizers involves trying to replicate the substances that naturally create the skin's matrix. Structural lipids attempt to do this. A substance called ceramide is an integral part of the skin's mortar. Ceramides themselves are too expensive to make available, so the cosmetic companies created a class of molecules known as "pseudo-ceramides" and put those in moisturizers. Another tactic is to incorporate into moisturizers such proteins as collagen, keratin and elastin, all of which are found naturally in the skin. It's not a bad idea in theory, but in practice, these protein molecules are too big to be easily absorbed into the skin. Instead, they end up filling the gaps in the stratum corneum, leaving behind a protective layer that also serves to smooth wrinkles.

To be a good moisturizer, the product should have all three of these ingredient categories to help maintain and restore your skin's barrier.

MOISTURIZERS FOR THE BODY

- Aveeno Eczema Care Moisturizing Cream and Daily Moisturizing Lotion
- Avène TriXéra+ Selectiose Emollient Balm
- Bioderma Atoderm PP Baume
- CeraVe Moisturizing Cream and Moisturizing Lotion
- Cetaphil Moisturizing Cream, Moisturizing Lotion and Restoraderm Replenishing Moisturizer
- La Roche-Posay Lipikar Baume AP+

MOISTURIZERS FOR THE BODY—NATURAL ALTERNATIVES

- Dr. Roebuck's Pure Body (contains vitamin E and lavender, which can be allergenic, as well as an essential oil called neroli oil, likely for its scent)
- Sunflower seed oil
- Virgin coconut oil

MOISTURIZERS FOR THE FACE

- Avène Tolèrance Extrême Cream
- La Roche-Posay Toleriane Ultra

MOISTURIZERS FOR THE FACE—NATURAL ALTERNATIVES

- Dr. Roebuck's Pure facial moisturizer—kudos to the company for creating a product with just seven ingredients. Finally, a natural alternative without 20 added botanicals!

Want a minimal chance of reaction to your makeup? Follow these rules.

1. When possible, use cosmetics with fewer than 10 ingredients.
2. Choose fragrance-free brands, such as:
   - Almay
   - Clinique
   - Marcelle
3. Watch out for brands that say "fragrance-free" but contain fragrance in the form of many added botanicals.
4. Powder cosmetics are better, as they don't need to be preserved.
5. Use black coloured mascara and eyeliner.
6. Avoid liquid eyeliner. Instead, use pencils.
7. Avoid mica or shimmer in your makeup.
8. Select earth-tone eye shadows.
9. Use physical or mineral sunscreen ingredients in foundations.
10. Use formaldehyde-free nail polish—and avoid shellac.

MAKEUP REMOVERS

- Cetaphil Gentle Makeup Remover
- La Roche-Posay Toleriane Eye Makeup Remover
- Micellar cleansers (can be used to remove makeup)

Topical Antioxidants

Hot product segments and sloppy science go hand in hand. Topical antioxidants are such a popular segment that it seems as if a new one comes out every month. They have names like coenzyme 10, alpha lipoic acid, resveratrol, green tea, soybean steroids, superoxide dismutase and pomegranate. Yet for many of these new, mainly botanical, antioxidants, evidence of their effectiveness at reducing the appearance of skin aging is weak, and there's no evidence to suggest their effects are long lasting.

And the studies that *do* show benefits tend to be industry sponsored.

Better grounded in science are the anti-aging benefits of such topical antioxidants as vitamin C, B3, E or niacinamide. These antioxidants are important because their molecules are small, allowing them to penetrate the skin. Some studies show benefits from stable vitamin C in concentrations between 5 and 15 percent. Combining the vitamin C with vitamin E appears to boost the antioxidative effects. So if you're going to use an antioxidant, I'd suggest a vitamin C preparation in a 5 to 15 percent concentration. Even better if it includes vitamin E.

One final thing: The effectiveness of an antioxidant can decrease over time. Throwing vitamin C into a product doesn't mean it will still be there when the jar has been sitting on the shelf for months. So try to find something that advertises the product's stability over time.

Cell Signallers

Cell signallers are a group of substances intended to fight aging on a cellular level. There are many of these, and some are more effective than others. The synthetic, prescription-drug version of vitamin A, known as retinoic acid, is the most powerful and scientifically tested anti-aging product available, and even the weaker, natural forms of vitamin A can help fight aging. But vitamin A can irritate the skin. For people who find vitamin A too irritating, I suggest polypeptides and growth factors (discussed below), although they have less scientific evidence to back up their anti-aging claims.

Here's how vitamin A works: Its two naturally occurring forms—retinol and retinyl palmitate—are metabolized into retinoic acid in the skin, and then that retinoic acid binds with key skin receptors that spur the production of collagen and renew the skin's top layer. Essentially, retinoic acid triggers an exfoliative effect, which is why it's considered a chemical exfoliant. The two chemists who first discovered this effect on the skin, Albert Kligman and James Fulton at the University of Pennsylvania, intended that retinoic acid be used for acne—but they also noticed that the substance had a powerful ability to reduce the appearance of wrinkles and stretch marks. Today, many cosmetic companies that sell products based on vitamin A, including Retin-A, also intend them to repair sun-damaged skin.

Pregnant women shouldn't use Retin-A or its variations. It can make your skin more sensitive to the sun, and it can be tricky for those with sensitive skin because it can burn and irritate the skin.

Retinol, one of the natural forms of vitamin A, is less irritating. (I use it myself, but only three times a week because more frequent use tends to irritate my skin.) There are some good drugstore brands, including RoC Pro-Correct and SkinCeuticals, but both of these contain allergens and other irritants, including the retinol itself. So tread carefully.

Other ingredient categories that can help regulate the skin cells include growth factors and polypeptides. Growth factors have names like Epidermal Growth Factor EGF and Transforming Growth Factor TGF. The companies that sell such products claim that they trigger the skin's natural healing response to repair the effects of aging and sun damage. But it's not known whether growth factors in cosmetic creams are stable, can be absorbed or exert enough of an effect in the skin to affect aging.

The polypeptides are more interesting and have more science behind them. One of the most well known, with a trade name of Matrixyl, was made in a cosmetic chemical lab to help satisfy the growing anti-aging market. It consists of five peptides—known as a pentapeptide—and is the first modern protein designed to alter cellular functioning. Since its launch in 2000, many more protein peptides with anti-aging claims have been developed. One of the more recent, and the one that has garnered lots of interest, is the topical Botox-like peptide known as Argireline, or Snap-8. Again, though, the studies here are few, not well controlled and industry sponsored.

Alpha Hydroxy Acid

The family of alpha hydroxy acids is another type of chemical exfoliant. They're a broad category that can include compounds derived from many different natural sources, yielding citric acid (oranges, lemons), glycolic acid (sugarcane), lactic acid (milk) and tartaric acid (grapes). Whatever particular type of acid it is, the alpha hydroxy compound is spread on the skin, where it sloughs off the dead cells on the uppermost layer of the stratum corneum by dissolving the chemical bonds that keep the cells connected to one another. The resulting chemical exfoliation exposes the newer cells underneath. Alpha hydroxy acids were among the first anti-aging products available on the market. Numerous studies show that they can slow down the progress of aging and improve the appearance of sun-damaged skin by increasing collagen density. Alpha hydroxy acid can also be very useful for acne-prone skin. I like:

- Reversa Skin Smoothing Body Lotion (10 percent glycolic acid, for the body)
- Reversa Skin Smoothing Cream (8 percent glycolic acid, for the face)

To sum up my common-sense approach to minimalist skincare:

BODY

1. *Cleanse.* Every regimen begins with some sort of cleansing.
    Remember, even the most minimalist and hardcore still shower
    and clean their body with friction. To wash with the minimum
    of interventions into your skin's natural function, I'd avoid
    conventional soap and suggest a syndet bar from my list—or use
    any of the syndet-type body washes without fragrance. Unless
    you've been rolling around in the mud, wash only underarms,
    groin and feet in the shower.

2. *Moisturize.* No one *needs* to use moisturizer; I don't think it's an
    integral part of a beauty regimen. But it can be helpful as we age.
    It can also be helpful for those who live in cold, dry climates, and
    for those with such skin disorders as atopic eczema and
    psoriasis. Remember, though, that if you have normal skin and
    you don't overwash, you might be able to forgo the moisturizer.
    If you're over the age of 30 and your skin has been damaged by
    the sun, then use a moisturizer that contains alpha hydroxy acid,
    such as Reversa Skin Smoothing 10% Body Lotion.

FACE

1. *Sunscreen.* Use sunscreen every day. It's best to use a product
    from the companies I recommend, particularly when out in the
    sun between the hours of 11 a.m. and 3 p.m., as well as other
    times throughout the day when the UV index is high. Use an
    SPF 30 and higher. For daily use when not in the sun for long
    periods of time, it's okay to use moisturizer or makeup with
    sunscreen—preferably one with titanium or zinc. Never use
    tanning beds!

2. *Cleanse.* At night, cleanse your face to remove oils, dirt and

pollution as well as makeup. Use the cleanser of your choice, but remember that the best ones for your skin are low to no foaming, with no fragrance or dyes. And watch out for additional ingredients that aren't necessary and could have an irritating effect on your skin—such as botanicals.

3. *Moisturizing and anti-aging products.* Here are my recommendations, according to the time of day when they're applied.

Morning: Use a moisturizer product with an antioxidant to help fight the oxidation that occurs throughout the day from UV light and air pollution. Lightweight serums or gels work particularly well under sunscreens.

- La Roche-Posay Redermic C or C10 cream
- SkinCeuticals C E Ferulic serum
- Vivier Vitamin C+E serum
- any stable vitamin C preparation or combination of vitamin C and other antioxidants, such as coffee bean extract, resveratrol, niacinamide or white tea

Night: After your evening cleansing, apply one of the cell signallers—retinol, retinoic acid, Matrixyl or other polypeptides, growth factors—particularly if you're in your thirties or older. What you choose to use will depend on the extent of your sun damage and skin reactivity. Retinol and the prescription alternatives should be used if you can tolerate them, since they have the best science. If you have more reactive skin and can't tolerate the vitamin A products, try peptides and, if even that triggers a reaction, growth factors, which aren't as effective but will give you some anti-aging benefits with less chance of irritation. Finally, you can add an exfoliating moisturizer with AHA or BHA several times a week. This would be helpful particularly if your skin is oily or acne prone. I often recommend this category to people in their twenties.

- Olay Pro XDeep Wrinkle Retinol (retinol)
- Rapid Wrinkle Repair by Neutrogena (retinol)
- RoC Pro-Correct Retinol (retinol)
- SkinCeuticals Retinol 1% and 0.5% (retinol)
- Oil of Olay Regenerist line (polypeptides)
- Neocutis (growth factors)
- SkinMedica (growth factors)

Note: In an industry where novelty remains a major selling point, cosmetic companies change their product names frequently. If you can't find one of the products listed in this chapter—or the rest of the book— check out my website at producteliminationdiet.com.

The Future of Skincare

One of this book's subtexts involves showing how things have changed—comparing the way we used to care for our bodies with the way we do it now. Your great-grandparents likely began their lives at a time when it was common to bathe just once a week. *Their* great-grandparents were lucky to get that. Today many of us feel gross if we don't get in at least a daily shower. What would fascinate someone who lived a century ago is the overall amount of primping conducted now by even the most laissez-faire of industrialized humans today.

Looking to the future of skincare is an interesting endeavour in part because we're *living* the future of skincare. And our reality is about to become even stranger.

I'll get to that in a second. But first, one big thing that should change *today*: The skincare sector should be regulated better. Europe, which at last count has banned 1300 chemicals from personal-care products, is way ahead of us in this regard. Most people probably believe that the U.S. Food and Drug Administration is regulating what goes into personal-care products like lipstick, skin cream and shampoo. In fact, that's not the case at all. In the United States, the Food, Drug and Cosmetic Act of 1938 allowed cosmetic companies to police themselves—and nothing's changed in the 80 years since.

Meanwhile, dozens of new ways of treating the skin have evolved, many of them dependent on new substances, both natural and synthetic. The industry as a whole is a lot bigger and more complicated. More people are allergic, and increasing numbers of people are dealing with sensitive skin and other maladies. In North America, those who are allergic to fragrances remain uninformed of the chemicals that are in their skincare products, putting them at risk of a nasty reaction each time they try a new moisturizer or shampoo.

Hopefully, things will improve over the next few years. A pair of American senators, California's Dianne Feinstein and Maine's Susan Collins, introduced new legislation in 2015. Known as the Personal Care Products Safety Act, the legislation would, for the first time, give the FDA the responsibility of reviewing chemicals used in cosmetic products. Problem is, it's been stalled on the floor of the U.S. Senate ever since.

In Canada, the legislation isn't great either. Skincare products here fall under the Food and Drugs Act, which ensures that "no person shall manufacture, prepare, preserve, package or store for sale any cosmetic under unsanitary conditions." Great, that should be obvious. Skincare companies also have to ensure Health Canada that their products don't contain "toxins." Cosmetic ingredients are subject to the Canadian Environmental Protection Act, which maintains a long list of things that should not be in skincare. But the regulations could be strengthened. In 2016, the country's environmental watchdog called on the federal government to require companies to disclose more about the chemicals that comprise such ingredient-list placeholders as fragrance, parfum, aroma and flavour. "Those catch-all terms can conceal a range of potentially hazardous chemicals," environment commissioner Julie Gelfand told reporters in 2016.

So let's hope all that changes in the short term. At the very least skincare companies should be required to list fragrance components that are allergenic, the way the EU does. Misleading terms like "hypoallergenic" and "sensitive skin" need to be regulated. Botanicals could be better regulated. And finally, I'd like to see regulators in both Canada and the U.S. working with the academic dermatologists who track reactions to skincare products. Information about ingredient safety needs to come from organizations that aren't funded by industry and from experts who don't have potential conflicts of interest.

Science-Fiction Skincare

Some of the things happening at the intersection of science and skincare are remarkable. For example, a chemical engineering professor at MIT has invented a polymer designed to stay on the face like a mask. You "paint" on a layer of liquid polymer, add another coat and the result is a second skin made from a chemical called polysiloxane. It's invisible, and permeable so that your skin can still breathe, but it's able to tighten the appearance of the whole face—erasing wrinkles, obscuring acne scars, removing years from your appearance. It may also be able to treat pre-existing skin conditions, such as eczema or psoriasis. I said earlier in the book that I doubt we'll ever be able to invent a barrier better than human skin—but maybe a second skin that eliminates a decade from your appearance will prove to be just as good?

Some of the most intriguing work in anti-aging is happening with DNA repair enzymes. Which may work on a number of levels.

Superficially, these enzymes may be able to stave off the signs of aging and keep us all looking younger for longer. More importantly, they may also be able to repair sun damage and prevent the development of skin cancer.

Knowing why requires knowing a bit about the exact mechanism by which the sun damages the skin. Most of us are aware that sun exposure creates wrinkles and sun spots. That happens in a couple of different ways. When it shines directly on skin-cell DNA, the sun's UV radiation can create abnormal structures in dermal DNA that prevent it from replicating properly. UV radiation can also create free oxygen radicals that damage cell bodies known as nucleotides. Both events can lead to the creation of cancerous tumour cells, which can grow and spread around the body.

Thankfully, the body fights the damage the sun causes. Enzymes in the skin bind to the damaged DNA and neutralize it. The enzymes achieve two separate, beneficial ends: They repair the damage caused by the sun, preventing wrinkles and erasing sun spots, and they neutralize a process that could develop into skin cancer.

The trouble is, the enzymes don't repair *all* the damage. Worse, the skin's ability to repair the damage decreases as we age.

But what if a cream or lotion could boost the action of the skin enzymes? That's the hope of Beverly Hills dermatologist Ronald Moy, who maintains a cosmetic surgery practice and conducts research out of the University of Southern California.

Dr. Moy has attempted to synthesize the skin's natural repair enzymes. By applying these enzymes directly to the skin, he hopes to enhance its ability to repair the sun's DNA damage. One difficulty was getting these topically applied enzymes to penetrate deep enough to where DNA is active. (Remember, the skin cells in the stratum corneum tend to be dead. The challenge is to get the enzymes to reach the level where the skin cells remain alive and replicating.) Simply smearing a cream onto the skin sees the enzymes neutralized before they can be absorbed into the skin's deeper layers, where the sun damage is happening.

So Dr. Moy has encapsulated the enzymes into molecules known as liposomes—which form a bubble-like protective layer of fat around the enzyme. The enzyme-bearing liposomes get smeared onto the skin in a cream. They penetrate the skin, and when they reach a disturbance in the skin pH—a telltale sign of DNA damage—the liposomes burst, releasing the enzymes to repair or neutralize the damaged DNA.

The research remains experimental. Dr. Moy himself likes to tell an anecdote that saw him use his own enzyme preparation on his wife's sunburn. The burn, he claimed, declined perceptibly within the hour, and was completely gone the next day. "DNA repair enzymes work like a seamstress," Dr. Moy told one publication. "They find damaged DNA, cut it out and then patch it with undamaged DNA."

Such anecdotes are just the sort of thing product salespeople would say to peddle their wares. But small-scale clinical trials have borne out Dr. Moy's story, showing that liposome-encapsulated DNA repair enyzmes with names like photolyase, endonuclease V and OGG-1 significantly boost the skin's ability to repair sun damage and fight the development of cancerous cells. If large-scale clinical trials produce similarly promising results, we may be just a few years away from a time when we can go to the pharmacy for a cream that helps prevent skin cancer and erases sunburns.

Genomics

Now for something even more innovative. Throughout 2016, Olay, the Procter & Gamble–owned brand, spent millions to fund research on the genomics of aging—that is, the way our skin's tendency to age well or poorly depends on the genetic information we inherit from our parents. (A genome is the complete set of genetic information contained in your cells. It's what makes you unique—your green eyes, wide nose and even the age at which you're apt to develop crow's feet near your temples.) There's a big drive in medicine to use the information in the genome to better tailor medical therapies to the needs of the individual. Olay's initiative is borrowing from medicine's precision-based approach and applying it to the problem of perpetuating human beauty. In this effort it's working in conjunction with 23andMe, a California-based genetics company.

It's a fascinating project. As a dermatologist, I have a better sense than most that some people age better than others. I've seen 55-year-old Asian women who look as though they're in their early thirties. Some African women I know feature a similar 20-year gap between their biological age and the age they appear to be. And although it happens more rarely, some Caucasian and Hispanic women also manage to appear ageless without cosmetic surgery or the use of lasers.

The fact is, some people age better than others.

What Olay is exploring with its research is whether the people who age well tend to share key aspects of their genome. Does everyone who ages into their eighties *without* getting laugh lines share some common length of DNA? What about people who never end up getting double chins or forehead lines? And if that's the case, can this knowledge be used to create a product that provides similar benefits to the rest of us?

The effort began with something called the Multi-Decade and Ethnicities study. That started as a partnership between Olay, 23andMe and Harvard University dermatologist Alexa Kimball. The research effort began in 2012 with a group of several hundred women, ranging in age from 20 to 70 and in ethnicity from African to Caucasian, Hispanic and Asian. A panel studied the faces of these women and, without knowing their actual ages, guessed how old they were based exclusively on their appearance.

The study's next phase grouped together the women who looked significantly younger than their biological age. Olay principal scientist Frauke Neuser told one publication that these women had skin that "seems to defy the rules of aging. . . . They look 'ageless' compared to other women the same age, without having undergone a cosmetic procedure."

Then Olay joined forces with 23andMe to analyze the genomes of these and other "ageless" women—eventually bringing nearly 60,000 women into the study. Meanwhile, researchers surveyed them about their lifestyle and skincare habits to determine whether they could learn something about how their skincare regimens had influenced their skin aging.

The genetic analysis revealed a set of DNA that the companies called the "Methuselah genes"—a reference to an early Biblical figure, an ancestor of Noah, said to have lived 969 years. Numbering about 2000 in total, the genes dictate a series of biological processes that protect the skin against the effects of the sun. In most women, these genes become less effective with age. But in about 20 percent of African Americans, and 10 percent of women overall, the Methuselah genes never slow down. That's why these women look ageless—because their skin never stops protecting itself from the sun. (Note to self: Avoid the sun and wear sunscreen!)

Dr. Neuser takes pains to point out that genetics isn't destiny. She told one publication that you can still influence how well you age, drawing an analogy between this ability and a game of cards, in which it's possible to be dealt a good hand and still lose or a bad hand and still win: "It's not just about the cards but about the person playing them."

As a result of the research, Olay began looking into ways it could help *everyone's* skin behave the same way as the lucky ones with Methuselah genes. Along with 23andMe, Olay also launched a larger study, with more than 155,000 participants, that investigated which behaviours helped women become exceptional skin agers. That research revealed that women who "almost always" wore protective sunscreen were 78 percent more likely to look younger than their biological age. The research also revealed that women who displayed a "positive attitude toward themselves" were 30 percent more likely to look younger than their biological age. (Although with that one, it's difficult to tease out which is cause and which is effect—rather than positivity somehow helping the skin, isn't it more likely that you feel positive toward yourself *because* you're an exceptional ager?)

Regular exercise, getting eight or more hours of sleep a night and high self-rated health were also among the predictors of youthful-looking skin. "In this study," said Dr. Neuser, "having skin that looks exceptionally young—ageless—was not down to luck; genetics plays some role, but factors within women's control have larger effects."

The major cosmetic companies are paying close attention to the genetics of skincare. One day soon, a visit to the cosmetic counter may begin with a DNA test. Then, based on your genetic information, the skincare retailer may be able to offer products tailored precisely for your DNA, creating an entire skincare strategy to follow for decades to come. The same test may also one day produce a comprehensive list of substances that could provoke an allergic or irritant skin reaction, helping you avoid those substances before such a reaction ever occurs. Or perhaps this genetic information will help predict when the various stages of aging will affect you—you'll get age spots *here*, deal with sagging *there*—and then work to counteract the problems. Presumably, Olay and its competitors will come up with the appropriate products to assist you along the way.

Designer Dermatology

Or perhaps you'll be able to splice from your genome the skincare problems you're destined to encounter—with gene-editing tools that are becoming more sophisticated with each year that passes.

Ever heard of CRISPR? It's a technique that allows scientists to *edit* a genome. The use of CRISPR to alter the genome of any living thing is controversial for all the usual ethical reasons—with playing God leading to some terrible *Jurassic Park* scenario where genetically designed creatures run amok. Nevertheless, in the short term, CRISPR has already been used by researchers at Rutgers University to attempt to create tougher wine grapes and better grass for golf courses. Chinese researchers have employed the technique to knock out genes related to growth hormones in pigs, yielding genetically engineered micro-pigs that may one day be sold as pets. Conversely, Chinese scientists also have used the technique to engineer extra-large goats.

Some biotechnology companies already plan to use CRISPR on humans—for example, to neutralize an inherited eye disease so that affected embryos will never become blind adults. Could CRISPR be used for comparatively trivial applications, like designing humans with sun-damage-battling Methuselah genes that never slow down? What about skin that never gets dry—or too oily? Programming the genome for higher cheekbones? A differently shaped nose? To be taller? With longer legs?

To hear some genetic engineers tell it, we're just a few decades away from being able to design most aspects of human appearance. There's something off-putting about that notion. After all, dealing with the various benefits and disadvantages of our appearance is part of the human condition. Once we're able to design every aspect of the way we look, will we retain the same peculiarly human vulnerability that characterizes us today? The possibility does raise some intriguing prospects, though. How exactly *will* everyone look when we can look however we want? And how will fashion trends affect things? Perhaps one year we'll all be wearing our ears long and tipped, à la Spock. Another season, and perhaps we'll prefer shorter earlobes—and longer noses will be in vogue.

Back to the Microbiome

One form of cosmetic-counter swabbing that could happen sooner rather than later concerns your skin's microbiome, which may contain as many clues about your skin health as your DNA. Analysis of the skin swab could provide data about the number, density and type of bacteria hosted by the skin. In turn, that information could provide a portrait of skin health. A behind-the-cosmetic-counter microbial expert might tell you that you need more of X and a little less of Y. Perhaps the expert will disappear into a lab somewhere, custom-design a blend of microbes just for you and then reappear moments later with a misting spray designed to address your microbiome's particular needs.

Before we get to that future, let's step back and recognize how far we've come. I recently took my youngest son to an astrophysics lecture at the University of Toronto. We learned all about the planets, and I was blown away by how tiny our solar system was compared to the rest of the universe. After, I asked the astrophysics professor how bacteria ever colonized our planet—bacteria being one of the first steps in the evolutionary chain that leads to humanity, and, actually, me sitting here working on this book you're reading.

"You know what?" the prof said. "That's one thing we don't know."

That's fascinating because bacteria are becoming one of the focal points of medicine—a hot topic that will dominate medical research for decades to come. My profession has speculated for years that bacteria played a role in conditions like eczema or psoriasis. But the more we learned about the microbiome, the more we grew to understand that it's not the *presence* of bacteria that may trigger such conditions, but an *imbalance* in the types of bacteria that exist on the skin.

This book has arisen in part because of that developing understanding—because dermatologists like me are just starting to understand that the way we take care of our skin may be playing havoc with the microbiome, which in turn may play a role in the increasing prevalence of numerous skin conditions. And that a better approach to skincare is needed to allow the microbiome to regulate itself. In fact, if you've reached this point in the book, you'll realize that our modern lifestyle has been an assault on the friendly germs living on us and in us.

The beauty industry is grasping the same thing. Which is why innovative products coming out of the personal-care product space are intended to return the skin's microbiome to a more balanced state.

For example, Teruaki Nakatsuji and Richard Gallo of the University of California, San Diego, recently published a fascinating study that could bring us closer to a novel non-medicated treatment for eczema. It all has to do with the interplay between a pair of bacteria on our skin. Nakatsuji and Gallo knew that the skin of people struggling with eczema tends to host large amounts of a bacteria called *S. aureus*. One theory is that these are somehow involved in causing eczema's symptoms—the dry, inflamed skin and itchy reaction.

To fight *S. aureus*, the two researchers swabbed the skin of people with eczema and, from the swabs, cultured a certain type of bacteria that inhibited the growth of *S. aureus*. That fought it off. Once they had enough of the *good* bacteria, which tended to belong to such strains as *S. epidermidis* or *S. hominis*, they blended the strains into a skin cream and slathered it onto the eczema. And the concentration of the bad bacteria, the *S. aureus*, dropped by 90 percent. Further studies are required to confirm that such a drop improves eczema symptoms.

But it's profoundly exciting stuff. Today we treat eczema with topical anti-inflammatory creams and antibiotics designed to rid the skin of bad bacteria. As well as some of the good. Those broad-spectrum antibiotics are like big bombs—they destroy all the microbes in an area.

In future, we'll fight such maladies with snipers. We'll be a lot more precise. We won't destroy all the microbiome, either. Rather, we may use good bacteria to selectively pick off just the bad bacteria. And to do that, we'll actually apply bacteria to the skin. It's a completely different approach from before.

Dermatologists and researchers have come up with numerous other ways to use bacteria to promote skin health. Many readers may be familiar with probiotics, which are products intended to encourage the development of a healthy microbiome. Most probiotics I've seen are meant to encourage a healthy *gut* microbiome—but over the next few years we'll also see ones that encourage a healthy *skin* microbiome.

Studies across the world are investigating which bacteria fight which skin conditions. One study showed that a *Lactobacillus plantarum* cream reduced skin redness and pimple size in people with acne. Similarly promising results happened for another type of bacteria, *E. faecalis SL-5*, which, just to be upfront about the therapy's grossness, was cultured from human feces. There's another type of bacterial product that's also the subject of tons of research: lysates, which aren't actually living bacteria but rather just the parts of them—dead bacteria, their cell walls, the things they create. Basically they're like fertilizer for germs. And they've been found to boost skin health in all sorts of ways. For example, the lysate of one bacteria was found to raise ceramide levels. Another improved sensitive skin.

Then there's AOBiome. That's the company I mentioned in Chapter 3. It was one of the first to market live bacteria–containing beauty products. And as I write this, AOBiome is busily working with several leading dermatologists on a whole host of academic studies designed to prove the effectiveness of its ammonia-oxidizing microbes.

One study explores how the ammonia-oxidizing bacteria affect keratosis pilaris, a common skin condition that sees the protein keratin creating small hard bumps on the skin, mostly in children and teens; the company's bacteria decreased the papule number by 45 percent compared to placebo. Another study investigates the bacteria's effects on eczema, and one of the most promising looks into its effect on acne. The benefits are logical enough. Recall that AOBiome's products are designed to return the skin microbiome to its natural state—to a naturally diverse microbiome the skin evolved to host. The same microbiome that exists in some of the world's most isolated tribal communities. Who, as you might remember from Chapter 3, don't suffer from acne.

The most intriguing research AOBiome is conducting grew out of the acne studies. When the company's live bacteria–containing mist was sprayed on the face, researchers noticed that its subjects experienced decreased blood pressure. The effect increased with higher doses of the mist.

That's remarkable. Something as simple as spraying germ-containing mist onto the skin actually decreased blood pressure. It sounds bizarre. But it also makes a lot of sense.

Many people have a grandparent with angina, which is chest pain that ensues when too little blood flows to the heart muscle. One treatment for that is nitroglycerine pills. The approach works because the body converts nitroglycerine to nitric oxide, which diffuses into the smooth muscle tissue that regulates the blood vessels. The blood vessels dilate, making it easier for the heart to pump and blood to flow through the body to the muscles of the heart. The same nitric oxide also plays a role in regulating inflammation.

Similarly, one byproduct of the ammonia-oxidizing bacteria's function on human skin is, you guessed it, nitric oxide. You sweat, the bacteria react with the ammonia in the sweat, leaving behind as a byproduct nitric oxide, which in turn gets absorbed into the body—possibly with the same effect as the nitroglycerine pills.

All told, AOBiome's research is helping to establish how powerful the skin microbiome can be. We used to fight skin disease by wiping out bacteria on the skin. In future, it's looking like we'll do just the opposite. That we'll fight skin disease by slathering bacteriological cultures onto our skin, in a skin cream, lotion or mist, the application of which is intended to return the microbiome to its healthy equilibrium.

Summing Up

I think these biome-enhancing products represent exciting progress. The research is a reflection that the dermatological research community, and the personal-care products sector over-all, are grasping the importance of the skin microbiome. The microbiologists I interviewed for this book agree that the skin microbiome of people in industrialized countries tends not to be as diverse as that of people from pre-industrialized communities. Will returning the microbiome to its previous diversity, similar to the one that exists on the skin of the Yanomami hunter-gatherers of the Amazon, entail an overall increase in skin health? At this stage, no one knows for sure. Exactly how our reduced bacterial

diversity has affected skin health will be investigated by researchers in the next decade, and beyond.

But one thing appears to be certain: Our modern lifestyle
has affected the skin's microbiome and impeded the skin's barrier
function. Consequently, we need to rethink the parts of that
lifestyle that are most damaging to the skin—the daily washing of
the entire body and our tendency to apply, often several times a
day, a host of skincare products with long ingredient lists that
include potential allergenic and irritant substances.

I've shown you the research that allergy, asthma and eczema
sensitive skin have increased in prevalence since we developed our
mania for cleanliness. I think that mania needs to be rethought.
Basically, we need to come to a *new and better clean*. I'm all for
fighting the transmission of communicable diseases with effective
handwashing and sanitizing. But excessive body and hair washing has
more to do with cultural norms and nothing to do with public health.

Remember, we lived for millions of years without doing much of
anything to the stuff that covers our bodies. And then, in the last
70 years or so, we began intervening. Weekly bathing turned to daily
showering, and then daily shampooing and daily all-over washing,
plus the many other ways we cleanse our faces, hands and the rest of
our bodies. Many of my female clients apply several dozen different
products to their bodies through the course of a given day.

It may be difficult for many people to grasp that soaping the
entire body every time you shower is bad for the skin. After all, as
Valerie Curtis pointed out in Chapter 2, being clean is in our genes.
So how to proceed? Always sanitize your hands. Cleanse your body
less frequently. When you're in the shower or bath, remember that
water is a great solvent. Most times the only places that really need
washing are your bits—and when you do wash them, use cleanser,
not soap. When it comes to products, less is more. And remember
that sun avoidance and sunscreen are the cornerstones of

anti-aging—and may be all the skincare you need, particularly if you're the proud owner of those Methuselah genes.

I'll leave with one final thought. One of the hottest market segments in the personal-care industry is natural and organic products. As I've pointed out throughout the book, these often contain botanical ingredients that can set up their users for allergic or irritant reactions. But rather than using more products, whether organic or synthetic, what could be more natural than leaving the skin of the body to care for itself?

Acknowledgments

This book came about from my desire to help my patients. I don't think I would have thought of the idea without their encouragement. I learn from you all every day in my office and I want to thank you.

I also want to thank my expedition team for that day in the tent at the North Pole when we discussed what we wanted to accomplish in the next 10 years. The experience led me to voice my desire to write this book, and then Shaun Francis put me in touch with Chris Shulgan. Thank you Shaun. Chris, you took my ramblings, rantings and many crises of faith and transformed them into a beautiful thing. It still amazes me to hear my own words told in such a readable and approachable way. You are a gifted writer and can take complex medical ideas and explain them so well. Thank you from the bottom of my heart.

To my editor at Penguin Random House, Andrea Magyar, thank you for taking me on and helping to shape the book with all your experience. You made it easy. But even some of the best books never reach their audiences. So thank you to the Penguin marketing and publicity teams, who toil mostly unrecognized and yet whose hard work is so crucial to the book's success. The same is true of my literary agents, the Cooke McDermid Agency, in particular my own agent, Chris Bucci.

To my mentor, Dr. Melanie Pratt, who first introduced me to contact dermatitis and all those crazy chemical ingredient names when I was a resident in dermatology. Over and above your incredible medical acumen in everything allergy-related, you are a beautiful soul who has always supported and encouraged me. Thank you to you, and to Dr. Joel Dekoven, for taking the time to read several chapters and offer up your knowledge. Dr. Sharon Jacobs gave the entire text a close read and offered numerous helpful suggestions.

Thank you to the numerous academics and researchers for contributing your time in interviews, and the wonderful research you've conducted that has contributed to this book's message: Dr. Sally Bloomfield, Dr. Howard Maibach, Dr. Michael Surette, Dr. Jack Gilbert, Dr. Apostolos Pappas and Dr. Spiros Jamas.

To my dermatology colleagues, those who trained me and who continue to teach me, thank you. I am so grateful to my friends who have supported me throughout this process by providing support and helping in numerous ways: Marlo Sutton, Carmen Sorger, Dr. George Sorger, Brent Sherman, Ciara Hunt.

Thank you to my wonderful boys and extended family for your support and understanding while I went through this incredibly challenging but rewarding process of writing a book—and who still can't believe it because "you can't even spell, Mom!" Brandon, Ryan and Spencer, Drew, Allie and Barclay. To Alex Kotyck, thank you for your support and desire to see me succeed, which is not always the way of the world.

Notes

INTRODUCTION

"In 2016, the U.S. Food and Drug Administration . . ." Study citation is
Michael Kwa, Leah J. Welty and Shuai Xu, "Adverse Events Reported
to the US Food and Drug Administration for Cosmetics and Personal
Care Products," *JAMA Internal Medicine* (2017).

"Or consider what's been happening . . ." Professor Michael Cork, head of
academic dermatology at the United Kingdom's University of
Sheffield, has conducted some excellent research on eczema, its
growing prevalence and the possible explanations. Valuable context
and statistics provided by Jonathan I. Silverberg and Jon M. Hanifin,
"Adult Eczema Prevalence and Associations with Asthma and Other
Health and Demographic Factors: A US Population–Based Study,"
Journal of Allergy and Clinical Immunology 132.5 (2013): 1132–1138.
Additional context provided by J. P. McFadden, "The Great Atopic
Diseases Epidemic: Does Chemical Exposure Play a Role?" *British
Journal of Dermatology* 166.6 (2012): 1156–1157.

"This epidemic troubles . . ." Dr. Howard Maibach wrote the book on
sensitive skin—literally, having co-authored the 2006 textbook
Sensitive Skin Syndrome. The Maibach quote is from E. Berardesca,

M. Farage and H. Maibach, "Sensitive Skin: An Overview,"
International Journal of Cosmetic Science 35.1 (2013): 2–8. The
Kligman quote is from A. M. Kligman et al., "Experimental Studies
on the Nature of Sensitive Skin," *Skin Research and Technology* 12.4
(2006): 217–222. The Kligman study also provides some of the
statistics cited in the following paragraph.

"Reports suggest . . ." Remaining statistics are from Miranda A. Farage and
Howard I. Maibach, "Sensitive Skin: Closing In on a Physiological
Cause," *Contact Dermatitis* 62.3 (2010): 137–149.

CHAPTER ONE

"When I discuss the situation . . ." Sugar statistics drawn from Rich
Cohen's *National Geographic* cover story in the August 2013 issue,
titled "Sugar Love: A Not-So-Sweet Story."

"If you recognize yourself . . ." The sensitive-skin scale is found in Laurent
Misery et al., "A New Ten-Item Questionnaire for Assessing Sensitive
Skin: The Sensitive Scale-10," *Acta Dermato-Venereologica* 94.6 (2014):
635–639. Used with permission.

CHAPTER TWO

"The trick is to differentiate . . ." The writing of Sally Bloomfield and
Graham Rook, and the International Scientific Forum on Home
Hygiene, informed my thinking on the difference between
hygiene and cleanliness. Particularly useful, and the source of the
quote, was R. Stanwell-Smith, S. F. Bloomfield and G. A. Rook,
"The Hygiene Hypothesis and Its Implications for Home
Hygiene, Lifestyle and Public Health," International Scientific
Forum on Home Hygiene (2012). Also see Sally F. Bloomfield et
al., "Time to Abandon the Hygiene Hypothesis: New Perspectives
on Allergic Disease, the Human Microbiome, Infectious Disease
Prevention and the Role of Targeted Hygiene," *Perspectives in
Public Health* 136.4 (2016): 213–224.

"The genus *Homo* first evolved . . ." The material on the evolution of the
human species, and the skin, is drawn from Yuval Noah Harari's book
Sapiens: A Brief History of Humankind. Penguin Random House, 2014.

"So how did we develop . . ." Valerie A. Curtis's work on the relationship
between human disgust and disease-avoiding behaviour is fascinating
and forms the basis for much of my material here. One good starting
point is "Dirt, Disgust and Disease: A Natural History of Hygiene,"
Journal of Epidemiology & Community Health 61.8 (2007): 660–664.

"Disgust of dirt is a part of human nature . . ." Unfortunately, it appears
that the BBC has archived the survey created by Valerie Curtis on the
BBC website. Last time I accessed it, I was only able to get two slides
in. Perhaps the BBC will reconsider. If that's the case, the latest URL
was http://www.bbc.co.uk/science/humanbody/mind/surveys
/disgust/index_2.shtml.

"So when did we start to *wash*?" Valerie Curtis's work informs this paragraph
and the one following on the development of human hygiene behaviour.
Babylonian society's use of soap dating to 2800 BCE is well documented.
One interesting source on the history of soap is Tejas P. Joshi, "A Short
History and Preamble of Surfactants," *International Journal of Applied
Chemistry* 13.2 (2017): 283–292.

"As Curtis points out . . ." Curtis, "Dirt, Disgust and Disease," p. 662.

"Indoor plumbing was common . . ." One of the most interesting books I
encountered researching this book was Geoffrey Jones, *Beauty
Imagined: A History of the Global Beauty Industry*. Oxford University
Press, 2010. Particularly fascinating was Chapter 3, "Cleanliness and
Civilization," from which much of this material is drawn.

"It would take several hundred more years . . ." The quote is taken from
Judith Walzer Leavitt in a review of Irvine Loudon's book *The Tragedy
of Childbed Fever* (Oxford University Press, 2000), *The New England
Journal of Medicine* 343.8 (2000): 587. The source for most of the
Semmelweis material is a 1983 English translation of "The Etiology,
Concept, and Prophylaxis of Childbed Fever" by Ignaz Semmelweis,

taken from Carol Buck's *The Challenge of Epidemiology: Issues and Selected Readings*. Semmelweis published the essay in 1858. Many other accounts of the rise of germ theory informed my account.

"Aristocrats who lived . . ." Much of the information here is drawn from Mark Tungate, *Branded Beauty: How Marketing Changed the Way We Look*. Kogan Page Publishers, 2011.

"Before germ theory came along . . ." Quote is from Jones, *Beauty Imagined*, p. 72.

"It took a series of wars . . ." Quote is from Jones, *Beauty Imagined*, p. 73.

"A 2012 paper . . ." R. Stanwell-Smith, S. F. Bloomfield and G. A. Rook, "The Hygiene Hypothesis and Its Implications for Home Hygiene, Lifestyle and Public Health," International Scientific Forum on Home Hygiene (2012).

"Well into the 20th century . . ." Ibid.

"The firm that did the most . . ." My visit to Procter & Gamble's world headquarters in Cincinnati informed much of the material in this section, with special thanks to the director of the P&G Heritage and Archives, Shane Meeker.

"Another innovation was the marketing . . ." Jones, *Beauty Imagined*, p. 75.

"Both Lever and P&G advertised heavily . . ." Ibid, p. 78. Much of the material in the following paragraphs is drawn from Jones's book, as well as Katherine Ashenburg's wonderful *The Dirt on Clean: An Unsanitized History*, Knopf Canada, 2007. Also informing my account was Sarah Everts, "How Advertisers Convinced Americans They Smelled Bad," *Smithsonian*, August 2, 2012. http://www.smithsonianmag.com /history/how-advertisers-convinced-americans-they-smelled-bad -12552404. Last accessed August 29, 2017. Also: Sarah Zhang, "How 'Clean' Was Sold to America with Fake Science," *Gizmodo*. February 12, 2015. http://gizmodo.com/how-clean-was-sold-to-america-1685320177. Last accessed August 2, 2017.

"By the dawn of the 20th century . . ." The relationship between the soap and advertising industries is fascinating and well documented, as is the role of one of the ad industry's most prominent female copywriters, Helen Lansdowne Resor, who created the Woodbury's Facial Soap campaign. For one fascinating account, see Kathy Peiss, *Hope in a Jar: The Making of America's Beauty Culture*. University of Pennsylvania Press, 2011.

"The market was growing..." The statistic is from Peiss, *Hope in a Jar*, p. 50.

"According to a July 2014 survey..." Euromonitor International, "Personal Appearances: Global Consumer Survey Results on Apparel, Beauty and Grooming." July 2014. For another interesting look at shower frequency, check out Olga Khazan, "How Often People in Various Countries Shower," *Atlantic Monthly* (2015): 1686–1687.

CHAPTER THREE

"Acne is nearly as prevalent..." A useful source of acne statistics was K. Bhate and H. C. Williams, "Epidemiology of Acne Vulgaris," *The British Journal of Dermatology* 168 (2013): 474–485.

"What's the prevalence of acne..." The material on Schaefer and the Okinawans is drawn from the 2002 *Archives of Dermatology* study mentioned two paragraphs later. The actual citation is Loren Cordain et al., "Acne Vulgaris: A Disease of Western Civilization," *Archives of Dermatology* 138.12 (2002): 1584–1590.

"The average adult human body..." The Grice and Segre study that was the source for this paragraph is Elizabeth A. Grice and Julie A. Segre, "The Skin Microbiome," *Nature Reviews Microbiology* 9.4 (2011): 244–253.

"So how does sensitive skin..." The Maibach-edited book is Enzo Berardesca, Howard L. Maibach and Joachim W. Fluhr, eds., *Sensitive Skin Syndrome*. CRC Press, 2006.

"The incidence of eczema..." Among the studies from which I drew context for the material on eczema and other skin maladies in this chapter was Sophie Nutten, "Atopic Dermatitis: Global Epidemiology and Risk Factors," *Annals of Nutrition and Metabolism* 66.Suppl. 1 (2015): 8–16, as well as Ramyani Gupta et al., "Time Trends in Allergic Disorders in the

UK," *Thorax* 62.1 (2007): 91–96. Also see Eric L. Simpson et al.,
"Emollient Enhancement of the Skin Barrier from Birth Offers Effective
Atopic Dermatitis Prevention," *Journal of Allergy and Clinical
Immunology* 134.4 (2014): 818–823. And Joseph A. Odhiambo et al.,
"Global Variations in Prevalence of Eczema Symptoms in Children
from ISAAC Phase Three," *Journal of Allergy and Clinical Immunology*
124.6 (2009): 1251–1258.

"We're accustomed to thinking . . ." One article that profoundly
influenced my thinking on the microbiome was Michael Specter's
New Yorker essay, "Germs Are Us," published in the October 22,
2012, issue. http://www.newyorker.com/magazine/2012/10/22
/germs-are-us.

"Lots of research has . . ." Hand microbiome statistics drawn from Noah
Fierer et al., "The Influence of Sex, Handedness, and Washing on the
Diversity of Hand Surface Bacteria," *Proceedings of the National
Academy of Sciences* 105.46 (2008): 17994–17999.

"When I went to medical school . . ." The Dr. Jack Gilbert quote is from
Carrie Arnold, "Rethinking Sterile: The Hospital Microbiome,"
Environmental Health Perspectives 122.7 (2014): A182–A187.

"But then in the 1980s . . ." The fact that hay fever was so rare that doctors
had a hard time finding cases to study is drawn from a pamphlet put
out by Sally Bloomfield's International Scientific Forum on Home
Hygiene. The hay fever statistics are drawn from the World Health
Organization's *White Book on Allergy 2011–2012*. The American
statistic is from the American College of Allergy, Asthma and
Immunology. The Canadian stat is from the Allergy/Asthma
Information Association.

"In 1989, a British epidemiology . . ." The landmark "hygiene hypothesis"
paper is David P. Strachan, "Hay Fever, Hygiene, and Household
Size," *BMJ: British Medical Journal* 299.6710 (1989): 1259.

"However, the body does . . ." For a good explanation of the "old friends"
line of thinking, see G. A. W. Rook, Charles L. Raison and C. A.

Lowry, "Microbial 'Old Friends', Immunoregulation and Socioeconomic Status," *Clinical & Experimental Immunology* 177.1 (2014): 1–12.

"Today we don't encounter . . ." The phrase "the right kind of dirt," which I love, comes from S. F. Bloomfield, R. Stanwell-Smith and G. A. Rook, "The Hygiene Hypothesis and Its Implications for Home Hygiene, Lifestyle and Public Health: Summary," International Scientific Forum on Home Hygiene (2012).

"To form the microbiome . . ." The J&J study is Kimberly A. Capone et al., "Diversity of the Human Skin Microbiome Early in Life," *Journal of Investigative Dermatology* 131.10 (2011): 2026–2032. The *Immunity* study is Tiffany C. Scharschmidt et al., "A Wave of Regulatory T Cells into Neonatal Skin Mediates Tolerance to Commensal Microbes," *Immunity* 43.5 (2015): 1011–1021.

"And that could also compromise . . ." The Grice and Segre quotes are from Elizabeth A. Grice and Julie A. Segre, "The Skin Microbiome," *Nature Reviews Microbiology* 9.4 (2011): 244.

"That said, from a scientific . . ." Ibid.

"Whereas the skin surface is . . ." The CDC paper is Elaine Larson, "Hygiene of the Skin: When Is Clean Too Clean?" *Emerging Infectious Diseases* 7.2 (2001): 225.

"Soaps and detergents . . ." Ibid.

"Possibly among the most . . ." The triclosan paper is Alyson L. Yee and Jack A. Gilbert, "Is Triclosan Harming Your Microbiome?" *Science* 353.6297 (2016): 348–349.

"Recently, a team from . . ." The Dorrestein research is chronicled in Paul Tullis, "The Man Who Can Map the Chemicals All Over Your Body," *Nature* 534.7606 (2016): 170–172.

"Another study conducted . . ." The Dorrestein study mentioned here is Amina Bouslimani et al., "Molecular Cartography of the Human Skin Surface in 3D," *Proceedings of the National Academy of Sciences* 112.17 (2015): E2120–E2129.

"Erika von Mutius, a German pediatrician . . ." Erika von Mutius, "The
    Microbial Environment and Its Influence on Asthma Prevention in
    Early Life," *Journal of Allergy and Clinical Immunology* 137.3 (2016):
    680–689. The northeastern Finland study is Tari Haahtela, "What Is
    Needed for Allergic Children?" *Pediatric Allergy and Immunology* 25.1
    (2014): 21–24.

"In a textbook . . ." The essay is David R. Whitlock and Martin Feelisch,
    "Soil Bacteria, Nitrite and the Skin," *The Hygiene Hypothesis and
    Darwinian Medicine.* Birkhäuser Basel, 2009. 103–115.

"Many dermatologists continue . . ." The "overwashing epidemic" quote is
    from Lily Talakoub, "Hair Washing—Too Much or Too Little?"
    Dermatology News, March 10, 2014. http://www.mdedge.com
    /edermatologynews/article/80893/aesthetic-dermatology/hair
    -washing-too-much-or-too-little. Last accessed August 29, 2017.

"I'm not the only one . . ." The story of AOBiome comes from the
    company's own website as well as Julia Scott, "My No-Soap,
    No-Shampoo, Bacteria-Rich Hygiene Experiment," *The New York
    Times Magazine,* May 22, 2014. https://www.nytimes.com/2014/05
    /25/magazine/my-no-soap-no-shampoo-bacteria-rich-hygiene
    -experiment.html. Last accessed August 31, 2017. Also from Kate
    Lunau, "I Skipped Showering for Two Weeks and Bathed in Bacteria
    Instead," *Motherboard,* June 17, 2016. https://motherboard.vice.com
    /en_us/article/78k4n4/showering-and-bathed-in-bacteria
    -instead-mother-dirt-aobiome-microbiome. Last accessed
    August 31, 2017.

"Sensing an opportunity . . ." The AOBiome quote is from the website of
    its subsidiary, Mother Dirt, located at http://motherdirt.com/mother
    -dirt-results-what-to-expect. Last accessed August 31, 2017

"A journalist named Julia . . ." From Scott's *New York Times Magazine* piece.

"Through Mother Dirt . . ." The company president's quote is from Lunau's
    piece in *Motherboard,* cited above.

"I recently spoke. . ." Jamas, personal interview.

"The non-industrialized cultures . . ." Loren Cordain et al., "Acne Vulgaris: A Disease of Western Civilization," *Archives of Dermatology* 138.12 (2002): 1584–1590.

CHAPTER FOUR

"I don't wonder about . . ." Information in this paragraph drawn from Bioderma's own corporate literature.

"Bioderma got its start . . ." Much of the background about Bioderma and its competitors is drawn from my communications with numerous different company employees through the course of my visit to the corporate headquarters, as well as my own background knowledge of the skincare industry.

"Through that experience . . ." P&G's "Science Behind" Symposium happened in early May 2016.

"Taking a brand and . . ." The material about Howard Moskowitz is drawn from Malcolm Gladwell's 2004 TED talk, "Choice, Happiness and Spaghetti Sauce," posted online at https://www.ted.com/talks/malcolm_gladwell_on_spaghetti_sauce, as well as Gladwell's *New Yorker* article "The Ketchup Conundrum," published in the September 6, 2004, issue. http://www.newyorker.com/magazine/2004/09/06/the-ketchup-conundrum. Both sources last accessed August 31, 2017.

"What underpinned its strategy . . ." The quote and sales data are from P&G's 2014 annual report, located online at https://www.sec.gov/Archives/edgar/data/80424/000008042414000057/fy201410kannualreport.htm. Last accessed August 31, 2017.

"In a *Harvard Business Review* article . . ." The article from which I've drawn much of the data in this paragraph is Bruce Brown and Scott D. Anthony, "How P&G Tripled Its Innovation Success Rate," *Harvard Business Review* 89.6 (2011): 64–72. Also see the *Harvard Business Review*'s interview with Anthony, "Inside P&G's Growth Factory," published on YouTube on July 6, 2011, at https://www.youtube.com/watch?v=_yVlXRTMxpE. Last accessed August 31, 2017.

"The result of this . . ." For more on the way P&G innovated to create the success of Febreze, check out Charles Duhigg's story in *The New York Times Magazine*, "How Companies Learn Your Secrets," February 16, 2012. http://www.nytimes.com/2012/02/19/magazine/shopping -habits.html. Last accessed August 31, 2017.

"I'll get to that . . ." Details on P&G's sale of its beauty brands to Coty drawn from Serena Ng and Ellen Byron, "P&G Exits Slumping Beauty Business," *The Wall Street Journal*, July 10, 2015. A1. The story values the sale of the brands to Coty at $13 billion, but movement in share prices would later value the deal at $12 billion. Details of P&G's CEO transition drawn from Ellen Byron et al., "Lafley to Hand Over Reins at P&G," *The Wall Street Journal*, July 28, 2015, B1.

"Heid seemed really receptive . . ." The website P&G launched to provide information about preservatives is located at http://us.pg.com/our -brands/product-safety/ingredient-safety/preservatives.

"Recall that beauty products . . ." Global skincare market information from Michelle Skelly, "How Consumers Shop: Anti-Aging Skin Care Market Trends 2015," LinkedIn, November 17, 2015. https://www.linkedin.com /pulse/how-consumers-shop-anti-aging-skin-care-market-trends -michelle-skelly. Last accessed August 31, 2017. The book is Geoffrey Jones, *Beauty Imagined: A History of the Global Beauty Industry*, Oxford University Press, 2010.

"And it got that way . . ." That P&G was the world's largest advertiser is from Nathalie Tadena, "P&G Eyes Big Ad Agency-Related Savings," *The Wall Street Journal*, October 23, 2015.

"While the scale of . . ." Jones, *Beauty Imagined*, p. 1.

"Such practices started from . . ." An interesting article on the origin of the term "soap opera" is Allie Leeds, "How Soap Operas Got Their Name; Why Are Soaps Called Soaps?" *ThoughtCo.*, May 8, 2016. https://www.thoughtco.com/how-soap-operas-got-their-name -3022985. Last accessed August 31, 2017.

"According to a 2017 survey . . ." Statistics on the amount spent on beauty are drawn from the SkinStore's 2017 customer survey, "How Much Is Your Face Worth? Our Survey Results Revealed!" Undated. http://www.skinstore.com/blog/skincare/womens-face-worth-survey-2017. Last accessed August 31, 2017.

"Still, it sounds about . . ." The first quote is from Janna Zittrer, "Facing Forward," *The Globe and Mail*, October 20, 2016. https://beta. theglobeandmail.com/life/fashion-and-beauty/beauty/why-the-mens-makeup-market-is-hotter-thanever/article32454404. The Vismay Sharma quote is from Katie Morley, "Male Cosmetics Counters Could Hit Department Stores in Five Years, L'Oreal Boss Says," *The Telegraph*, August 6, 2017. http://www.telegraph.co.uk/news/2017/08/06/male-cosmetics-counters-could-hit-department-stores-five-yearsloreal. Last accessed August 31, 2017.

CHAPTER FIVE

Note: Much of the information in this chapter is drawn from publications by the North American Contact Dermatitis Group. Learn more about the NACDG on their website, located at https://www.contactderm.org.

"How many potential . . ." Find the Environmental Working Group survey at "Why This Matters—Cosmetics and Your Health," *EWG's Skin Deep Cosmetics Database*, April 12, 2011. http://www.ewg.org/skindeep/2011/04/12/why-this-matters/#.WYx1uHeGPpA. Last accessed September 4, 2017.

"Then, for reasons that . . ." The article is Rachel Abrams, "Growing Scrutiny for an Allergy Trigger Used in Personal Care Products," *The New York Times*, January 23, 2015. https://www.nytimes.com/2015/01/24/business/allergy-trigger-found-in-many-personal-care-items-comes-under-greater-scrutiny.html. Also see Ohio State University Wexner Medical Center, "Got an Itch? Allergy to Moistened Wipes Rising, Says Dermatologist," *ScienceDaily*, March 3, 2014. http://www.sciencedaily.com/releases/2014/03/140303083204.htm. Both last accessed September 4, 2017.

"Today, in contact dermatitis . . ." The contact allergen of the year is published
    annually in the medical journal *Dermatitis*. For more information, see Mari
    Paz Castanedo-Tardana and Kathryn A. Zug, "Methylisothiazolinone,"
    Dermatitis 24.1 (2013): 2–6. For details of the disturbing reaction, see
    Mary Beth Quirk, "There's a Preservative That Can Give You an
    Awful, Itchy Rash—And It's Probably in Your Bathroom,"
    Consumerist, July 20, 2015. https://consumerist.com/2015/07/20
    /theres-a-preservative-that-can-give-you-an-awful-painful-rash-and
    -its-probably-in-your-bathroom. Last accessed September 4, 2017.

"Many companies do try . . ." The survey of products marketed to those
    with sensitive skin is Carsten R. Hamann et al., "Is There a Risk Using
    Hypoallergenic Cosmetic Pediatric Products in the United States?"
    Journal of Allergy and Clinical Immunology 135.4 (2015): 1070–1071.

"Up to 10 percent of . . ." The stat that about 10 percent of the population
    will react to a cosmetic product comes from a press release from the
    American Academy of Dermatology, "Allergies: Culprit Could Be in
    Cosmetic Bag," March 11, 2000. https://www.newswise.com/articles
    /allergies-culprit-could-be-in-cosmetic-bag.

"Here, then, are the NACDG's most current . . ." The NACDG publishes
    this information every several years or so. This information is taken
    from the most recent publication of top allergens in the years 2013–
    2014: Joel G. DeKoven et al., "North American Contact Dermatitis
    Group Patch Test Results 2013–2014," *Dermatitis* 28.1 (2017): 33–46.

"The stuff is big . . ." The quote is from Amy Verner, "Why Your Shampoo
    Smells So Good," *Elle (Canada)*, December 1, 2015. https://www
    .pressreader.com/canada/elle-canada/20151201/281719793450440
    . Last accessed September 4, 2017.

"The trouble is that . . ." The description of oakmoss's scent is drawn from
    Courtney Humphries, "Engineering Replacements for Essential
    Perfume Ingredients," *Wired*, October 21, 2011. https://www.wired.com
    /2011/10/ff_perfume. Learn more about the International Fragrance
    Association at http://www.ifraorg.org.

"Pragmatically speaking . . ." Allergen prevalence data drawn from Joel G.
DeKoven et al., "North American Contact Dermatitis Group Patch
Test Results 2013–2014," *Dermatitis* 28.1 (2017): 33–46.

"And more fragrances are being . . ." For the mechanics of the working of
fragrance, and general trends in the fragrance industry, I drew on the
writing of the wonderful Zoe Diana Draelos, specifically her article,
"How Fragrance Technology Irritates Sensitive Patients," *Dermatology
Times*, December 1, 2014. http://dermatologytimes.modernmedicine
.com/dermatology-times/news/how-fragrance-technology-irritates
-sensitive-patients. Last accessed September 1, 2017.

"That said, the fragrance . . ." The actual EU cosmetic legislation is EU
Cosmetics Directive 76/768/EEC. Annex III of EU Cosmetic
Regulation 1223/2009 currently lists 26 allergens, all of which must be
included in the ingredients list on the label or packaging of a product
if they are present in concentrations greater than 0.001% in leave-on
products and 0.01% in rinse-off products. Learn more at https://
ec.europa.eu/growth/sectors/cosmetics/legislation_en.

"The EU labelling restrictions . . ." The Canadian federal government
report is located on the website of the Office of the Auditor General
of Canada, "Report 3—Chemicals in Consumer Products and
Cosmetics," March 31, 2016. Located online at http://www.oag-bvg
.gc.ca/internet/English/att___e_41394.html. For further context and
quotes, I'm grateful to Margo McDiarmid, "Cosmetics and
Household Products Need More Safety Oversight, Watchdog Says,"
CBC News, May 31, 2016. http://www.cbc.ca/news/politics
/environment-watchdog-spring-report-2016-1.3608675.

"Many of us recall . . ." That formaldehyde was classified as a carcinogen in
2011 is found at "Formaldehyde," National Institute of Environmental
Health Sciences, https://www.niehs.nih.gov/health/topics/agents/
formaldehyde/index.cfm. Last accessed September 4, 2017.

"Frequently known as MDBGN . . ." That in 2005 the EU banned the use
of MDBGN in leave-on products is, like much of the information on

EU Cosmetics Directive 76/768/EEC, drawn from the EU website on the legislation, found at https://ec.europa.eu/growth/sectors /cosmetics/legislation_en and last accessed September 4, 2017.

"After fragrances and preservatives . . ." For information about paraphenylenediamine, I drew on Vanessa Ngan, "Allergy to Paraphenylenediamine," *DermNet New Zealand*, undated. https:// www.dermnetnz.org/topics/allergy-to-paraphenylenediamine. Last accessed September 4, 2017.

"Also gaining popularity as . . ." To learn more about alkyl glucosides, see Denis Sasseville, "Alkyl Glucosides: 2017 Allergen of the Year," *Dermatitis* 28.4 (2017): 296.

"What the lip balm *did* contain . . ." Learn more about reactions to EOS lip balm products, and resultant class-action lawsuits against the company, in Greg Seals, "EOS Lip Balm Lawsuit Updates: The Brand Is Compensating Customers Who Experienced Blisters and Rashes," *Glamour*, November 2, 2016. https://www.glamour.com/story/eos-lip -balm-lawsuit-blisters-compensation. Learn more about allergic reactions to natural skincare products, and find the source of the NPD group stat, in Anna Wilde Mathews, "Surprise Allergies to 'Natural' Skin-Care Products," *The Wall Street Journal*, April 18, 2016. https://www.wsj.com /articles/surprise-allergies-to-natural-skin-care-products-1460999491 ?mod=e2tw. Both articles last accessed September 4, 2017.

"The problem is that . . ." The Italian study is M. Corazza et al., "Use of Topical Herbal Remedies and Cosmetics: A Questionnaire-Based Investigation in Dermatology Out-Patients," *Journal of the European Academy of Dermatology and Venereology* 23.11 (2009): 1298–1303.

"In 2016, *The Wall Street Journal* . . ." That article is Anna Wilde Mathews, "Surprise Allergies to 'Natural' Skin-Care Products," *The Wall Street Journal*, April 18, 2016. Link above.

"Commonly known as 'bee glue' . . ." Source of the quote about propolis is G. A. Burdock, "Review of the Biological Properties and Toxicity of Bee Propolis (Propolis)," *Food and Chemical Toxicology* 36.4 (1998): 347–363.

"Ask most people about . . ." One of the first dermatological articles on the harmful influence of water on human skin comes from Isaac Willis, "The Effects of Prolonged Water Exposure on Human Skin," *Journal of Investigative Dermatology* 60.3 (1973): 166–171.

"As cut-and-pasted from . . ." To check out Abundance Naturally Baby Balm yourself, see the company's website, located at https://www .abundancenaturally.com/product/abundance-naturally-baby-balm. Note that the explanations for each ingredient had changed slightly the last time I accessed the page on September 4, 2017.

"Many essential oils can . . ." The quote about essential oils is from Rose Ann Gould Soloway, "Essential Oils: Poisonous When Misused," *Poison Control: National Capital Poison Center,* undated. From the website of George Washington University Medical Center's National Capital Poison Center. http://www.poison.org/articles/2014-jun /essential-oils.

"The condition, which features . . ." The article is Laurent Misery et al., "Sensitive Scalp: Does This Condition Exist? An Epidemiological Study," *Contact Dermatitis* 58.4 (2008): 234–238.

CHAPTER SIX

"Her case was one . . ." Learn more about reactions to EOS lip balm products, and resultant class-action lawsuits against the company, in Greg Seals, "EOS Lip Balm Lawsuit Updates: The Brand Is Compensating Customers Who Experienced Blisters and Rashes," *Glamour,* November 2, 2016. https://www.glamour.com/story/eos -lip-balm-lawsuit-blisters-compensation.

CHAPTER SEVEN

"In 2014, I joined . . ." Learn more about the North Magnetic Pole Expedition and True Patriot Love's many other worthy endeavours at http://truepatriotlove.com.

"Let's pause a moment . . ." Ashenburg, *The Dirt on Clean,* pp. 260-261.

"Today, according to a . . ." For showering frequency in developed and
   other nations, see Olga Khazan, "How Often People in Various
   Countries Shower," *The Atlantic*, February 17, 2015. https://www
   .theatlantic.com/health/archive/2015/02/how-often-people-in
   -various-countries-shower/385470. Last accessed September 1, 2017.
"People love the shower." The CDC quote is from Elaine Larson,
   "Hygiene of the Skin: When Is Clean Too Clean?" *Emerging Infectious
   Diseases* 7.2 (2001): 225.
"But it's still perfectly . . ." The Woodcock quote is from Rebecca
   Voelker, "Say Goodbye to Some Antibacterials," *JAMA* 316.15 (2016):
   1538–1538. The 1600 figure for the number of different products sold
   in Canada that may contain triclosan is from the Government of
   Canada's fact sheet "Triclosan—Questions and Answers,"
   Chemical Substances, last modified March 20, 2012. http://www
   .chemicalsubstanceschimiques.gc.ca/fact-fait/triclosan-eng.php#a9.
   Last accessed September 4, 2017.
"The sheer volume of . . ." The quote is from Zoe Diana Draelos,
   "Considerations for Hair Washing Frequency," *Dermatology Times*,
   August 18, 2014. http://dermatologytimes.modernmedicine.com
   /dermatology-times/content/tags/cosmeceuticals/considerations
   -hair-washing-frequency. Last accessed September 1, 2017.
"Co-washes usually use . . ." For more on WEN, see "FDA Information for
   Consumers About WEN by Chaz Dean Cleansing Conditioners,"
   U.S. Food & Drug Administration, May 9, 2017. https://www.fda.gov
   /cosmetics/productsingredients/products/ucm511631.htm. Last
   accessed September 1, 2017.
"Hand cleansing can be . . ." CDC information on handwashing is on the
   organization's website. "When & How to Wash Your Hands," Centers
   for Disease Control and Prevention, March 7, 2016. https://www.cdc.gov
   /handwashing/when-how-handwashing.html. Last accessed
   September 1, 2017.
"'The goal,' according to . . ." Quote is from Elaine Larson, "Hygiene of

the Skin: When Is Clean Too Clean?" *Emerging Infectious Diseases* 7.2 (2001): 225.

"But if your hands . . ." The WHO quote is from "Alcohol-Based Handrub Risks/Hazards," World Health Organization, undated. http://www. who.int/gpsc/tools/faqs/abhr2/en. Last accessed September 1, 2017.

CHAPTER EIGHT

"And I am not . . ." The atopic dermatitis prevalence quote is from Michael Cork, "Preventing Atopic Dermatitis by Changing the Way We Treat a Newborn's Skin from Birth," Expert Forum: Neonatal Skin Health and Skin Care Symposium, September 12, 2015. The review is a summary of the presentations at the symposium.

"These are anecdotal accounts . . ." For a summary of the AAD position, consult Tara West, "How Often Should You Bathe a Child? Why Doctors Say You Should Stop Giving Your Kid a Bath Every Night," *Inquisitr*, February 10, 2016. http://www.inquisitr.com/2783926/how -often-should-you-bathe-a-child-why-doctors-say-you-should-stop -giving-your-kid-a-bath-every-night. Last accessed September 1, 2017.

"Another consideration is . . ." The quote, and much of the information in this chapter about the processes affecting an infant's skin soon after birth, are drawn from Joanne Kuller, "Development of the Neonatal Skin Microbiome," Expert Forum: Neonatal Skin Health and Skin Care Symposium, September 12, 2015. The review is a summary of the presentations at the symposium.

"In fact, the early . . ." More information on the Dominguez-Bello microbiome swabbing is found at Ewen Callaway, "Scientists Swab C-Section Babies with Mothers' Microbes," *Nature*, February 1, 2016. https://www.nature.com/news/scientists-swab-c-section-babies- with-mothers-microbes-1.19275. Last accessed September 1, 2017.

"Nearly 20 years of . . ." The Cork article "Preventing Atopic Dermatitis . . ." referenced above was useful, as was the Kuller article from the same expert forum.

"Once you're through the . . ." The paper is J. P. McFadden, "The Great
    Atopic Diseases Epidemic: Does Chemical Exposure Play a Role?"
    British Journal of Dermatology 166.6 (2012): 1156–1157. Atopic dermatitis
    statistics drawn from S. K. Bantz, Z. Zhu and T. Zheng, "The Atopic
    March: Progression from Atopic Dermatitis to Allergic Rhinitis and
    Asthma," *Journal of Clinical & Cellular Immunology* 5.2 (2014): 202.

"Lots of studies have . . ." More on the role of filaggrin in atopy is found in
    Shuai Xu et al., "Cost-Effectiveness of Prophylactic Moisturization for
    Atopic Dermatitis," *JAMA Pediatrics* 171.2 (2017): e163909–e163909.
    The McFadden article cited above also has some good material on
    filaggrin.

"But which one?" See the Cork article referenced above for his account of
    the experiment.

"Because of such studies . . ." The 2015 study is Carsten R. Hamann et al.,
    "Is There a Risk Using Hypoallergenic Cosmetic Pediatric Products
    in the United States?" *Journal of Allergy and Clinical Immunology* 135.4
    (2015): 1070–1071.

"We've known this for . . ." The study pertinent to this book is Andrea
    Sherriff, J. Golding and Alspac Study Team, "Hygiene Levels in a
    Contemporary Population Cohort Are Associated with Wheezing
    and Atopic Eczema in Preschool Infants," *Archives of Disease in
    Childhood* 87.1 (2002): 26–29.

"In fact, the harmful . . ." See the guidelines at "How Often Do Children
    Need to Bathe?" American Academy of Dermatology, September 12,
    2016. https://www.aad.org/media/news-releases/how-often-do
    -children-need-to-bathe. Last accessed September 1, 2017. See further
    guidelines on bathing at "How Often Do Children Need a Bath."
    American Academy of Dermatology, undated. https://www.aad.org
    /public/skin-hair-nails/skin-care/child-bathing. And see the
    American Academy of Pediatrics' suggestions on healthy bathing of
    newborns at "To Bathe or Not to Bathe." Healthychildren.org,
    November 2, 2009. https://www.healthychildren.org/English

/ages-stages/baby/bathing-skin-care/Pages/To-Bathe-or-Not-to
-Bathe.aspx. Last accessed September 1, 2017.

CHAPTER NINE

"Then there's the other . . ." For more on Robert Brumm's experience
    giving up soap, see his blog at www.robertbrumm.com/my-blog.

"Brumm's not the only one . . ." For more on soap-free living, see Jackie
    Hong, "Soap Free for Seven Years," *Toronto Star*, March 13, 2017.
    https://www.thestar.com/life/2017/03/13/soap-free-for-seven
    -years.html. Also see Cathy Bussey, "'I Haven't Used Shampoo in 2
    Years . . .,'" *The Telegraph*, August 12, 2014. http://www.telegraph.co.uk
    /women/womens-life/11021507/I-havent-used-shampoo-in-2-years
    -and-my-hair-has-never-looked-better.-Welcome-to-the-UKs-no
    -poo-movement.html.

"There's a good reason . . ." The source of my account of Tarnopolsky's
    experiments is Gretchen Reynolds, "Younger Skin Through Exercise,"
    The New York Times, April 16, 2014. https://well.blogs.nytimes.
    com/2014/04/16/younger-skin-through-exercise. Last accessed
    September 1, 2017.

"One of the world's . . ." For Krutmann's study, see Anke Hüls et al.,
    "Traffic-Related Air Pollution Contributes to Development of Facial
    Lentigines: Further Epidemiological Evidence from Caucasians and
    Asians," *Journal of Investigative Dermatology* 136.5 (2016): 1053–1056.

"It is not a problem . . ." My source on Krutmann's quote is Damian
    Carrington, "Air Pollution Causes Wrinkles and Premature Ageing, New
    Research Shows," *The Guardian*, July 15, 2016. https://www.theguardian
    .com/environment/2016/jul/15/air-pollution-causes-wrinkles-and
    -premature-ageing-new-research-shows. Last accessed September 1, 2017.

"U.K. cosmetic doctor . . ." Ibid.

"The process of glycation . . ." A fascinating paper about the relationship
    between diet and the skin, from which I've drawn much of the
    information in this section, is Rajani Katta and Samir P. Desai, "Diet

and Dermatology: The Role of Dietary Intervention in Skin Disease,"
The Journal of Clinical and Aesthetic Dermatology 7.7 (2014): 46.

"Then there's the most . . ." Source on the UVA-irradiated mice study, and
skin cancer, is the Katta and Samir paper, cited above.

"You might be tempted . . ." In general I found the writing of Zoe Draelos
to be tremendously helpful in the writing of this book. In particular,
the source for this paragraph's quote is "Can You Eat Your Way to
Healthy Skin?" Zoedraelos.com, undated. http://www.zoedraelos
.com/articles/diet. Last accessed September 1, 2017.

"The short answer is yes." The Australian study is Adèle Green et al.,
"Daily Sunscreen Application and Betacarotene Supplementation in
Prevention of Basal-Cell and Squamous-Cell Carcinomas of the Skin:
A Randomised Controlled Trial," *The Lancet* 354.9180 (1999): 723–
729. The 10-year follow-up that demonstrated that sunscreen prevents
melanoma is Adèle C. Green et al., "Reduced Melanoma After
Regular Sunscreen Use: Randomized Trial Follow-Up," *Journal of
Clinical Oncology* 29.3 (2010): 257–263.

"The ingredients that cosmetic . . ." For background on moisturizers,
I'm grateful to C. W. Lynde, "Moisturizers: What They Are and
How They Work," SkinTherapyLetter.com, 6:13. December 2001.
http://www.skintherapyletter.com/2001/6.13/2.html. Last accessed
September 1, 2017.

CHAPTER TEN

"Hopefully, things will improve . . ." For some useful context on the
situation in the United States, see Sheila Kaplan, "Cosmetics May
Face New Safety Regulation . . .," *Stat*, September 27, 2016. https://
www.statnews.com/2016/09/27/cosmetics-fda-congress-safety. Last
accessed September 1, 2017.

"In Canada, the legislation . . ." For a look at the situation in Canada, see
Margo McDiarmid, "Cosmetics and Household Products Need More
Safety Oversight, Watchdog Says," *CBC News*, May 31, 2016. http://

www.cbc.ca/news/politics/environment-watchdog-spring-report
-2016-1.3608675. The article was also the source of the quote. Last
accessed September 1, 2017.

"Some of the things . . ." Brooke Le Poer Trench, "The Future of Skin
Care," *Harper's Bazaar*, September 7, 2016. http://www.harpersbazaar.
com/beauty/skin-care/a16910/new-skin-care-innovations. Last
accessed September 1, 2017.

"But what if a . . ." I was introduced to the work of Dr. Ronald Moy in Judy
Johnson, "DNA Repair Enzymes: The Anti-Ageing Ingredient That Can
Undo Years of Damage," *Get the Gloss*, March 15, 2016. https://www
.getthegloss.com/article/dna-repair-enzymes-the-skincare-ingredient
-that-can-repair-years-of-damage. Last accessed September 1, 2017.

"The research remains . . ." The Dr. Moy quote is ibid.

"Now for something even . . ." Information about the Olay and 23andMe
partnership contained in "Olay Provides New Insights to the Age-
Long Nature versus Nurture Beauty Debate," P&G News Release,
January 19, 2017. http://news.pg.com/press-release/pg-corporate
-announcements/olay-provides-new-insights-age-long-nature-versus
-nurture-b. Last accessed September 1, 2017.

"The study's next phase . . ." Megan Cahn, "Are There Really Genes
That Make People Look Younger?" *Refinery29*, June 24, 2015.
http://www.refinery29.com/olay-study-younger-gene. Last
accessed September 1, 2017.

"Ever heard of CRISPR?" For more on CRISPR, see Michael Specter,
"The Gene Hackers," *The New Yorker*, November 16, 2015. http://
www.newyorker.com/magazine/2015/11/16/the-gene-hackers. Also
see Brooke Borel, "CRISPR, Microbes and More Are Joining the War
Against Crop Killers," *Nature*, March 14, 2017. http://www.nature.com
/news/crispr-microbes-and-more-are-joining-the-war-against-crop
-killers-1.21633. Both articles last accessed September 1, 2017.

"For example, Teruaki Nakatsuji . . ." Nakatsuji and Gallo's approach to
treating eczema is detailed in Ed Yong, "A Probiotic Skin Cream

Made with a Person's Own Microbes," *The Atlantic*, February 22, 2017.
https://www.theatlantic.com/science/archive/2017/02/a-personalized
-probiotic-skin-cream-made-with-a-persons-own-microbes/517473.
Last accessed September 1, 2017.

"Studies across the world . . ." A good overview of probiotics and
dermatology is Mary-Margaret Kober and Whitney P. Bowe, "The
Effect of Probiotics on Immune Regulation, Acne, and Photoaging,"
International Journal of Women's Dermatology 1.2 (2015): 85–89.

"The most intriguing research . . ." Much of AOBiome's exciting research
opportunities were described by Spiros Jamas during an interview we
conducted by telephone as research for this book. To learn more
about AOBiome's research into hypertension therapies, see the press
release "AOBiome Launches Phase 2 Clinical Trial Using Novel
Bacterial Platform for Treatment of Hypertension," AOBiome.com,
December 15, 2016. http://www.aobiome.com/news_
item&item=110&title=AOBiome-Launches-Phase-2-Clinical-Trial
-Using-Novel-Bacterial-Platform-for-Treatment-of-Hypertension.
Last accessed September 1. 2017.

*Note: Much of the material in this book is drawn from the background
knowledge I've accumulated in my own medical career as a practising
dermatologist and member of the University of Toronto's Faculty of Medicine.
Some of the rest is freely available on the web. This reference section is by no
means a comprehensive compilation of all my sources, but rather my effort to list
the most interesting or relevant of the references I used.*

Index

Note: Page numbers in italic indicate boxed text or an illustration.